Self-Assessment in Immediate Medical Care

T J Hodgetts
MB BS, MRCP (UK), DipIMC RCSEd
Captain, RAMC
British Military Hospital, Hannover

Baillière Tindall
London   Philadelphia   Toronto   Sydney   Tokyo

Baillière Tindall   24—28 Oval Road
W.B. Saunders   London NW1 7DX

The Curtis Center
Independence Square West
Philadelphia, PA 19106—3399, USA

55 Horner Avenue
Toronto, Ontario M8Z 4X6, Canada

Harcourt Brace Jovanovich Group Australia Pty Ltd
30—52 Smidmore Street
Marrickville
NSW 2204, Australia

Harcourt Brace Jovanovich Japan Inc
Ichibancho Central Building, 22—1 Ichibancho
Chiyoda-ku, Tokyo 102, Japan

© 1990 Baillière Tindall

ISBN 0—7020 1510—5

Typeset by Setrite Typesetters Ltd.

Printed and bound in Great Britain by MacKays of Chatham PLC, Chatham, Kent

British Library Cataloguing in Publication Data is available

Acknowledgements

The publishers would like to acknowledge the following for supplying
illustrations to be used in this book: Professor A.J. Camm (Pages 209,
211, 212, 214, 215, 217, 219, 221—225), Dr D. Ward (pages 210,
218—220, 227), Dr D.J. Rowlands (213, 228) and Laerdal Medical
(pages 229, 230).

Contents

Preface

"It is the mark of a mature mind to bear uncertainty with equanimity".

N. Colnet

How will you react in an emergency? What would you do for a man who collapses in the street in ventricular fibrillation or is trapped, injured, in his car? These things are not taught in medical school, but are among a junior doctor's greatest fears.

This book was sparked by the Diploma of Immediate Medical Care (Royal College of Surgeons of Edinburgh), a subject on which there are excellent text-books, but little, if anything, to aid revision by self-assessment. The exam includes a triage exercise (a concept which many doctors are unfamiliar with) and rhythm strip interpretation.

This book will be of use to anyone who wishes to assess, or further, their knowledge in the field of immediate pre-hospital and hospital care, but particularly those preparing for the Diploma examination and doctors or nurses involved in accident and emergency work. There are also important principles that any medical student will find useful. Some of the questions that I have set are intentionally contentious; I hope that they will stimulate further research and discussion among you.

I would like to thank Dr James Wright FRCP for his patience, interest and literary guidance.

TJH
Hannover

Multiple Choice Exercises

Basic Life Support
Trauma Life Support
Cardiac Life Support
Medical Emergencies
Miscellaneous

After each heading there are five related questions or statements (A–E). Decide whether they are true or false and record your response. The answers (T or F) are given at the top of the next page followed by some notes relating to the topic.

A precordial thump

A. Will deliver about 50 joules of energy.
B. Should be performed routinely at all cardiac arrests.
C. May be sufficient to restore sinus rhythm in ventricular fibrillation.
D. May convert ventricular fibrillation into asystole.
E. Is dangerous in complete heart block.

FFTTF

1. A precordial thump is a blow with a clenched fist over the junction of the middle and lower thirds of the sternum.
2. It delivers about 8 joules of energy.
3. It should be reserved for WITNESSED ventricular fibrillation or ventricular tachycardia as it is only effective if administered rapidly (15−20 seconds) after the dysrhythmia onset. Results are not consistent.
4. Ventricular fibrillation or tachycardia may be converted into asystole, or ventricular tachycardia into fibrillation; it is therefore potentially detrimental.
5. The heart rate in complete heart block can be maintained by regular, rhythmic precordial thumps ("fist pacing") while preparing for pacing.
6. Thumping is not a substitute for external chest compressions.
7. Thumping is not recommended in infants.

With expired air ventilation

A. The oxygen content is 21%.
B. Carbon monoxide poisoning will place the rescuer at risk.
C. The recommended ratio of ventilations to chest compressions is 2 : 15 for one rescuer.
D. The mouth is opened on exhalation with mouth-to-nose technique.
E. Dentures should always be removed.

1. Expired air ventilations (EAV) and external chest compressions (ECC) are the fundamentals of Basic Life Support — that is, life support with no equipment other than your own hands and brain.

2. The oxygen content of expired air is 16−17%, as compared with 21% atmospheric air.

3. EAV can be delivered through the patient's mouth (mouth-to-mouth) or nose (mouth-to-nose): the latter is more practical for those with a small mouth and may be more aesthetically appealing. With mouth-to-nose, the patient's mouth should be opened on exhalation to overcome the tendency to partial airway obstruction.

4. Do not remove a full set of well fitting dentures — these will support the mouth during EAV; any plates or partial dentures should, however, be taken out.

5. The correct ratio for ventilations to chest compressions is

   - ONE RESCUER   2 ventilations to 15 compressions
   - TWO RESCUERS   1 ventilation to 5 compressions

   (1 : 5 is also used with one rescuer resuscitating a neonate)

6. EAV to a patient with carbon monoxide poisoning will not place the rescuer at undue risk and should not be a reason for withholding resuscitation.

With external chest compressions

A. The correct depth is 1−2 cm in infants.
B. Compressions in adults should be at 80 per minute.
C. Each compression should be released rapidly.
D. Optimal compressions will sustain the brain for 20 minutes.
E. Coronary blood flow is 40% of normal.

1. Chest compressions are given with the heel of one hand placed two fingers breadth above the xiphisternum (or 2/3 of the way down a line between the suprasternal notch and the xiphisternum) and the other hand resting on this, with or without fingers interlocking. Compression is then produced through straight arms with the weight of the body directly over the patient's chest.

2. Incorrect hand position is not only inefficient, but may be dangerous:

   - TOO LOW   — xiphisternum may be forced into the liver or heart
                    — raised abdominal pressure produces regurgitation
   - TOO LATERAL   rib fractures
   - TOO HIGH   sternal fracture

3. The correct depth of compression is

   - Infants 1−2 cm
   - Children 2−4 cm
   - Adults 4−5 cm

   To avoid overcompressing, use only the heel of one hand in children and two fingers in infants (adjust the infant position to one finger breadth below the inter-nipple line).

4. The compression rate should be around 80 per minute for adults, but at least 100 per minute for small children and infants. With one rescuer, 60 compressions per minute will be achieved in the adult when remembering the time for interspersed ventilations.

5. Compression phase should be 50−60% of each cycle to maximize output.

6. With resuscitation in the most experienced hands, cerebral perfusion will be less than 30% and coronary perfusion only 5% of normal; an average brain will be sustained for approximately 20 minutes.

7. Closed chest compressions produce blood flow not only by direct compression of the heart between the sternum and vertebrae, but also by a rise in intrathoracic pressure ("thoracic pump").

The triple airway manoeuvre

A. Is head tilt + chin lift + mouth open.
B. Is suitable for a suspected cervical spine injury.
C. Is more effective than head tilt + neck lift in opening the airway.
D. Is best performed when kneeling to one side of the patient.
E. Is used when ventilating through a pocket mask.

FFTFT

1. The "triple airway manoeuvre" is head tilt + jaw thrust + mouth open.

2. The majority of airways (80%) are opened satisfactorily by head tilt + chin lift or head tilt + neck lift. In those whom these manoeuvres are not successful, additional jaw thrust is recommended.

3. It is best performed while kneeling behind the casualty's head. Both hands are used to lift the lower jaw forward (little fingers in angle of jaw) while opening the mouth with the thumbs. The base of the thumbs oppose the nostrils and pressure with the wrists on the forehead causes the head to extend.

4. This is a difficult manoeuvre to perform properly, made even more difficult if ventilations must be interspersed with the chest compressions and the rescuer has to kneel at the casualty's side.

5. A pocket mask (Laerdal) held over the mouth and nose in this way is the best method of ventilatory support in the absence of any airway device which isolates the trachea from the oesophagus (endotracheal tube; Brain laryngeal airway; pharyngotracheal lumen airway).

6. The triple airway manoeuvre is NOT, however, suitable for a suspected cervical spine injury when minimal head and neck movement is imperative: in this instance jaw thrust alone is used.

"New" CPR

A. Is the currently recommended method for cardio-pulmonary resuscitation.

B. Involves synchronous ventilations and chest compressions at 40 per minute.

C. Leads to a rise in carotid blood flow.

D. Is associated with an improvement in coronary blood flow.

E. Produces a better cerebral perfusion than standard techniques.

1. The term "New CPR" was first used by Chandra in 1980 and refers to synchronous ventilations and chest compressions at a rate of 40 per minute.
2. His work was experimental in dogs and endotracheal intubation was a prerequisite.
3. It is claimed that up to 90% of the pre-arrest carotid blood flow can be regained, but most of this is directed to the external carotids. This increased carotid flow is also at the expense of a diminished coronary flow.
4. There is a slight rise in systolic blood pressure, but a fall in diastolic pressure.
5. The intrathoracic pressure rises, impeding venous return from the head and neck which then raises the intracranial pressure and further impedes cerebral perfusion.
6. It does not seem sensible to recommend any method of resuscitation that leads to a fall in cerebral and myocardial perfusion.

In patients who are choking

A. Back blows are better than abdominal thrusts.
B. Abdominal thrusts should not be performed in children.
C. Abdominal thrusts produce higher airway pressures.
D. If they are conscious they should be encouraged to cough.
E. If they are unconscious they should receive abdominal thrusts.

1. There is considerable controversy between the relative efficacy of back blows and of abdominal thrusts ("Heimlich manoeuvre"). Neither should be taught to the exclusion of the other.

2. In the early 1970s Heimlich described the "champagne cork" effect of abdominal thrusts on a foreign body placed in beagles' tracheas. He also labelled back blows as "death blows". The thrust is believed to produce an "artificial cough" by forcing the diaphragm upwards.

4. Abdominal visceral damage is reported with the Heimlich manoeuvre and it is not recommended for use in children.

5. When the patient is conscious they should first be encouraged to cough and to lean forwards, allowing the foreign body to fall out with gravity.

6. When the patient is unconscious, abdominal or chest (similar to chest compression) thrusts should be given.

7. The sequence for a conscious choking victim is therefore:

    COUGH — 4 × BACK BLOWS — 4 × ABDOMINAL THRUSTS (then alternate blows and thrusts)

8. Greater success is likely with direct laryngoscopy and removal of the foreign body with Magill's forceps.

An oropharyngeal (Guedel) airway

A. Is inserted upside down.
B. Can cause laryngospasm.
C. Is better tolerated than a nasopharyngeal airway.
D. Alone will adequately support an unconscious (but breathing) patient's airway.
E. Correct size is gauged by the distance between the corner of the mouth and the earlobe.

TTFFT

1. Oropharyngeal (Guedel) airways are curved plastic or rubber tubes which splint the mouth open and hold the tongue forwards, away from the posterior wall of the pharynx.

2. The airway is inserted upside-down then rotated through 180 degrees: this prevents the tongue being pushed back as the airway is advanced.

3. Average adult sizes are 2 (female), 3 and 4 (male).

4. The correct size is otherwise an airway with a length equivalent to the distance between the corner of the mouth and the earlobe.

5. If the airway is too long it may impinge on the epiglottis and bend it over the laryngeal opening.

6. If the airway is too short it will not support the tongue.

7. Vomiting and laryngospasm can be induced in those with intact pharyngeal reflexes — these airways should therefore only be used in the deeply unconscious. A nasopharyngeal airway is better tolerated and can be used in the semiconscious.

8. The insertion of an oropharyngeal airway does *not* remove the need to maintain a proper head position — in particular, persistent head tilt is needed to prevent the airway from slipping out if the neck should flex.

The oesophageal obturator airway

A. Can still be used if the trachea is accidentally intubated.
B. Produces poor tidal volumes.
C. May cause oesophageal rupture.
D. Does not prevent aspiration of stomach contents.
E. Must be removed before endotracheal intubation.

FTTFF

1. The oesophageal obturator airway is an airway adjunct that has found some favour with American paramedics, but not with the emergency services in the United Kingdom.

2. It consists of a face mask, to which is attached a blind-ending tube perforated along the upper third of its length.

3. The airway is inserted blind into the oesophagus and a distal cuff then inflated to prevent regurgitation of stomach contents.

4. It is designed to be used by personnel not trained in endotracheal intubation, but its insertion is still an acquired skill. It is, however, no substitute for intubation.

5. Complications include

    - Tracheal intubation (up to 10%)
    - Oesophageal perforation
    - Promotion of vomiting, aspiration and laryngospasm on insertion if the patient is not deeply unconscious

6. Tidal volumes are poor.

7. It is not suitable for those under 16 years or the very short (its length precluding its use);

8. A modification, the oesophago-gastric tube airway (OGTA), is open-ended, allowing aspiration of stomach contents. Ventilation is via the nose.

9. Precautions must be taken to prevent aspiration on removing the device: either a cuffed endotracheal tube should be *in situ* or the patient should be breathing spontaneously.

Concerning airway adjuncts

A. 100% oxygen can be delivered through a pocket mask.

B. The Brook airway provides good tongue support.

C. The Brain laryngeal mask airway is unsuitable for use in infants.

D. Insertion of a pharyngo-tracheal lumen airway is dangerous when cervical cord damage is suspected.

E. The Safar airway allows ventilation through the nose or the mouth.

TFFFF

1. Any airway adjunct that removes the unpleasantness of mouth-to-mouth resuscitation holds an immediate attraction. Ideally, it should also provide good tongue support, offer little air flow resistance, be easy to insert and be cheap to buy.

2. The simplest device is a plastic sheet with a central bite block/viral filter (Resusciade; Life-Aid).

3. The pocket mask (Laerdal) removes the need for direct mouth-to-mouth contact and has an optional non-regurgitating disposable ventilation valve. Oxygen delivered at 30 litres/minute through the side port will equate to 100%. There is no tongue support — if ventilation (mostly through the nose) is inadequate, insert a Guedel airway.

4. The Brook airway is supplied as a "Professional" and "All Purpose" model; the latter has virtually no tongue support whilst that of the professional model is soft and flimsy. Resistance is high. Rescuer protection is provided by a non-return valve.

5. The Brain laryngeal mask was developed in 1983. It is available in four sizes (for infants to adults) and consists of an oropharyngeal tube that feeds into an inflatable cuffed spoon-shaped mask. The mask is wedged in the hypopharynx and prevents regurgitation while allowing adequate ventilation. Its appeal is that it can be inserted blind, quickly and without moving the head and neck.

6. The pharyngo-tracheal lumen airway shares the advantages of the Brain laryngeal mask: they are both suitable for pre-hospital use where endotracheal intubation is difficult (entrapment; cervical spine injury). Simply, it is two parallel tubes — a short tracheal and longer oesophageal tube. If these are accidentally transposed, an obturator is removed from the oesophageal tube and ventilation can proceed.

7. The Safar-S airway is a size 4 and a size 2 Guedel airway end-to-end. The Dual-Aid allows ventilation through the nose or the mouth.

Oxygen

A. Oxygen from a portable "D" size cylinder at 8 litres/minute will last 40 minutes.

B. Oxygen at 50% is dangerous after 6 hours.

C. Oxygen via nasal prongs is well tolerated at 10 litres/minute.

D. Delivery can be accurately controlled with a Venturi mask.

E. Oxygen through an MC or Hudson mask at 4 litres/minute will deliver 60%.

1. Oxygen has been available for medicinal use since the late 18th century (the gas was discovered by Priestly in 1772 and introduced shortly afterwards into England by Beddoes).

2. Standard cylinder sizes are:

Size	Capacity (litres)
D	340
E	680
F	1360

   A size "D" cylinder will therefore deliver 8 litres/minute for just over 40 minutes.

3. Inhalation of 100% oxygen (or anything over 80%) for more than 12 hours produces symptoms of respiratory tract irritation with cough, sore throat and nasal stuffiness, leading on to tracheobronchitis and pulmonary atelectasis. This does *not* occur with 50% oxygen. When oxygen is breathed at greater than atmospheric pressure, toxicity is first indicated by central nervous symptoms (muscle twitching and paraesthesia).

4. Accurate oxygen concentrations are best achieved using a Venturi mask, when air is entrained through holes in the mask with oxygen at a fixed flow rate. There are five available masks — 24%, 28%, 35%, 40% and 60%. Critical control of oxygen delivery is essential for chronic bronchitics, whose hypoxic drive will be abolished with a high oxygen concentration (use 24%).

5. Nasal prongs are comfortable with flow rates of 3−4 litres/minute: higher than this can cause nasopharyngeal mucosal ulceration and abdominal distension (from swallowed air).

6. A Hudson or MC (Mary Catterall) mask — that is, a standard face mask — will deliver approximately 40% oxygen at 4 litres/minute and 60% at 8 litres/minute.

Concerning intubation

A. Nasal intubation is less traumatic than oral.
B. Nasal intubation is contraindicated with a basal skull fracture.
C. The correct endotracheal tube size for a 6-year-old is 4 mm internal diameter.
D. In adults, the epiglottis should be pulled forward with the laryngoscope.
E. It can produce a dangerous rise in intracranial pressure.

FTFFT

1. Intubation is indicated to

   - Protect the airway from aspiration
   - Provide ventilatory support
   - Remove secretions

2. Endotracheal intubation is performed under direct vision of the vocal cords and requires some flexion of the neck and extension of the head ("sniffing the morning air" or "modified Jackson position"). This is **not** acceptable in the presence of a cervical spine injury when nasotracheal intubation, which requires less neck movement, is a preferable alternative.

3. Nasotracheal intubation is, however, traumatic to the nasal mucosa and brisk bleeding is not uncommon. It is contraindicated in suspected basal skull fractures.

4. The correct endotracheal internal tube diameter for children is calculated with the formula:

$$\frac{Age}{4} + 4\frac{1}{2} = \text{diameter (in millimetres)}$$

   Average adult sizes are 8.5−9.5 mm (male) and 7.5−8.5 mm (female). Nasal tubes are usually taken to be 1 mm smaller. Average adult lengths are 24 cm (male) and 22 cm (female): it is worth pre-cutting the commonly used sizes.

5. In adults a curved-bladed laryngoscope is used, with the tip of the blade placed in the vallecula between the tongue and the epiglottis. Straight-bladed laryngoscopes are customarily used in infants when the blade is placed over the epiglottis.

6. Upper airway stimulation with the laryngoscope will result in reflex hypertension and a rise in intracranial pressure — in the presence of brain injury this may lead to further oedema or haemorrhage.

Cricothyrotomy

A. Will provide an adequate airway for up to 6 hours.
B. Is performed just below the cricoid cartilage.
C. Is preferable to tracheostomy as a rapid airway procedure.
D. In children is best performed with a needle.
E. Complications include sub-glottic stenosis.

FFTTT

1. The cricothyroid membrane can be felt as a small depression between the thyroid and cricoid cartilages.

2. Cricothyrotomy will rapidly establish an airway when the upper respiratory tract is obstructed. It may be needed in

   - facial burns or trauma
   - anaphylaxis (e.g. bee/wasp sting)
   - infection (epiglottitis; Vincent's angina)
   - angio-oedema

3. The technical problems and risk of severe haemorrhage of tracheostomy are largely avoided; it is also much quicker.

4. Needle cricothyrotomy is performed with the largest-bore cannula to hand. The patient may exhale through a partially obstructed upper airway or else a second cannula is placed adjacently. This method is recommended for children: subglottic stenosis may be the result of damage to the cricoid cartilage by an excessive cricothyroid membrane incision. In the under 12s tracheal rings are unable to keep the trachea open against a negative inspiratory pressure. Only the cricoid ring at this age is strong enough and, therefore, damage to it may cause airway obstruction.

5. Commercial cricothyrotomy kits (Mini-Trach II) contain a guarded blade, 4 mm cannula with introducer and a securing ribbon tape.

6. Cricothyrotomy is only a temporary procedure, providing an adequate airway for less than an hour, after which time carbon dioxide retention will be problematic.

7. Additional oxygen can be delivered from a ventilating bag or by jet insufflation.

With a flail chest

A. The flail segment moves outwards on inspiration.
B. A sternal flail is the least stable.
C. Paradoxical chest wall movement may not be noticed for 12 hours.
D. Positive pressure ventilation is always advisable.
E. Should be strapped as a first aid measure.

FTTFT

1. A "flail chest" describes the paradoxical movement of a segment of the chest wall with respiration. This segment comprises a minimum of three ribs, each fractured in two places, or the sternum.

2. The mechanism behind the injury is crushing of the chest, as occurs against the steering wheel in a road traffic accident when the individual is not restricted by a seatbelt. Flail segments of the lateral chest wall are the commonest, but a sternal flail is the least stable.

3. The functional result is that the mediastinum moves to and for during respiration and air is exchanged across the carina between the lungs. Theoretically, if the flail segment were large enough, respiration would consist only of an oscillation of air between the two lungs ("pendelluft").

4. The flail segment itself may not be large enough to cause hypoxia, but associated chest pain from rib fractures will contribute to hypoventilation.

5. As a first-aid measure, the segment is splinted: the patient should be turned on the affected side and adhesive strapping applied. Strapping around the whole of the chest will impair ventilation on the unaffected side.

6. Analgesia, oxygen and vigorous respiratory care may be all that is required for small flail segments; for the patient who is cyanosed and respiratorily distressed, positive-pressure ventilation is needed.

7. Underlying injuries must be considered and a haemothorax/pneumothorax drained before positive pressure ventilation is started (lest it become a tension pneumothorax).

8. Deterioration of lung function and compliance secondary to lung contusion may unmask a previously missed flail segment up to 24 hours after the injury.

Tissue perfusion is monitored by

A. Capillary refill.
B. Pulse rate.
C. Urine output.
D. Core−surface temperature gradient.
E. Pulse oximetry.

TTTTT

1. In all forms of shock the tissue perfusion is inadequate for the needs of the tissue at the time. A simple assessment of improving tissue perfusion as a result of volume replacement in hypovolaemic shock is a falling pulse rate, decrease in anxiety or confusion and a capillary refill of under 2 seconds (on pressing the nail bed). Equally non-invasive is the monitoring of blood pressure, core—surface temperature gradient and oximetry. Invasive monitoring includes hourly urine output and central venous pressure.

2. One of the earliest indicators of deteriorating perfusion is an increase in the core—surface temperature gradient (thermister on big toe), since vasoconstriction is an early compensatory response, but this is not practical in pre-hospital care. A pulse oximeter will detect a fall in oxygen saturation measured peripherally by an infrared clip-on probe (finger/earlobe); the plethysmographic waveform will also alter. These machines *are* portable and battery powered.

3. Blood pressure is not a sensitive indicator of reduced blood volume in a fit adult: more than 1 litre of blood can be lost (normal adult volume is 5 litres) before the systolic pressure falls below 100 mmHg. The pulse rate is more predictive (and this, too, is displayed on a pulse oximeter).

4. Normal urine output is 40—50 ml/hour: with a blood loss of 1 litre this will fall to 20—30 mls and with 2 litres lost will be negligible.

When cross-matching blood

A. There is a minimum time of 25 minutes.
B. Group compatible blood can be available in under 5 minutes.
C. O negative blood carries no risk of sensitizing the patient.
D. An "urgent" cross-match will not test as extensively for antibodies.
E. At the road-side, a hospital identification number should be obtained.

1. There is no differrence in the technique between an "urgent" and a "routine" cross-match — "urgent" just identifies the sample to the laboratory to be processed immediately.

2. Serum cannot be withdrawn from the sample for centrifugation until the blood has clotted and retracted, a process which will take 2–5 minutes after the sample was placed in the bottle. 15 minutes is the minimum incubation time to perform a complete compatibility test to detect any abnormal antibodies. Along with the time to transport the blood to the laboratory, there is a minium time of 25 minutes to perform a cross-match.

3. Blood grouping can be done from an EDTA sample (bottle used for "full blood count") and group compatible blood issued within a few minutes.

4. 17% of the Caucasian population carry the Rhesus genotype CDe/CDe. When such a person is transfused with O-negative blood (genotype cde/cde) there is a risk of acquiring anti-c antibodies.

5. In view of the catastrophic consequences of a mismatched transfusion, every effort should be made to safeguard the patient against receiving the wrong blood. With mass casualties, there may only be a number on the request form to coincide with a number on the patient's forehead. In more conventional circumstances, it is reasonable of the laboratory to expect a hospital identification number: the details of a roadside (particularly entrapment) casualty can be radioed ahead and a hospital number can be available for when an urgent sample arrives.

Dextran

A. Dextran 40 has caused renal tubular necrosis.
B. Dextran 70 reduces platelet adhesiveness.
C. Administered volume is limited to 1 litre.
D. Dextran is only supplied in glass bottles.
E. Dextran should not be started until blood has been taken for cross-match.

1. Dextran is a fermentation product of sucrose by *Leuconostoc mesenteroides*. It is supplied as Dextran 40, 70 and 110; the number refers to the average molecular weight (40,000; 70,000; 110,000).

2. Dextran is stored in glass bottles, which are heavy and bulky to carry and impractical for pre-hospital use.

3. Dextran coats the red cell membrane and interferes with the cross-match: blood should be withdrawn before starting dextran (but if necessary the red cells can be washed).

4. Dextran increases coagulation times by impairing platelet function and fibrin formation.

5. Volume in resuscitation is limited to 1 litre.

6. Dextran 40 in excess produces a viscid urine which may extend to renal tubular obstruction with consequent "post-renal" failure.

7. Dextran is retained by the reticulo-endothelial system and slowly excreted (the half-life is measured in days).

8. There is a risk of allergic reactions.

9. As plasma expanders in hypovolaemic shock, dextrans have largely been replaced by Haemaccel and Gelofusine and it must remembered that they are CUMULATIVE, TOXIC and INTERFERE WITH COAGULATION.

Haemaccel

A. Will interfere with the cross-match.
B. Does not interfere with coagulation.
C. Will cause flocculation of citrated blood in the giving-set.
D. Has a shelf life of 2 years.
E. Allergic reactions are common.

FTTFF

1. Haemaccel is a straw-coloured, colloidal solution of poly-geline (degraded gelatin) with an average molecular weight of 35,000.

2. It is used to replace blood or plasma in hypovolaemic shock in a ratio of 1:1 Haemaccel to lost fluid. Up to 25% blood loss can be replaced by Haemaccel alone.

3. The shelf life is approximately 5 years.

4. In contrast with dextran

   - Allergic reactions are rare.
   - The cross-match is not interfered with.
   - There is no effect on coagulation.

5. Citrated blood should not be mixed with Haemaccel as the calcium ions in the colloidal solution will cause the blood to clot in the giving-set.

6. Haemaccel will gel below 3°C, but rewarming will reverse this; freezing does not alter its properties.

7. Gelofusine is very similar to Haemaceel, but contains less calcium (<0.4 mmol/litre compared to 6.25 mmol/litre) and more sodium (154 mmol/litre compared to 145 mmol/litre). Both will maintain the circulating blood volume for several hours (4−6 hours on average).

8. 6% Hetastarch (Hespan) is also a "plasma expander", but its effects can last in excess of 24 hours.

The "Trauma Score"

A. Correlates injuries with survival.
B. Incorporates an adjusted Glasgow Coma Scale.
C. Takes account of the pulse rate.
D. Has a maximum score of 100.
E. Can be used as a method of triage.

TTFFT

1. There is more than one numerical system which attempts to correlate injury with survival. Examples include the "Trauma Score" (Champion *et al.*) and the Maryland scoring system ("Injury Severity Score").

2. The Trauma Score has a maximum of 16 points, 16 implying virtually guaranteed survival while a score of less than 3 indicates irrecoverable injury.

3. The components of the Trauma Score are respiratory rate, respiratory effort (normal/retractive/none), systolic blood pressure, capillary refill (normal/delayed/none) and an adjusted Glasgow Coma Scale (maximum score = 5).

4. The Injury Severity Score quantifies the three most severely injured regions in terms of **minor** (score 1 point); **moderate** (score 2 points); **severe** — but non-life-threatening — (score 3 points); **severe** — life-threatening, but survival probable — (score 4 points); **critical** — survival uncertain — (score 5 points). The individual scores are SQUARED then ADDED together. The maximum score is 75 (virtually unsurvivable).

5. A scoring system is only useful if

   - It accurately predicts survival.
   - It is reproducible between different observers.
   - It is easy to apply (as a method of triage with mass casualities).

In hypovolaemic shock

A. Crystalloid is replaced 1 : 1 for lost blood.
B. Normal saline may produce an acidosis.
C. Hartmann's may produce an acidosis.
D. Whole blood is mandatory.
E. Blood pressure invariably falls with 25% blood volume loss.

1. "Shock" is inadequate tissue perfusion resulting in general-ized tissue hypoxia.

2. Hypovolaemia is one cause of shock, but the commonest encountered in trauma (others are SEPTIC, CARDIOGENIC and NEUROGENIC).

3. A crystalloid is a true solution, passing freely through a semipermeable membrane and can be crystallized. Examples include Hartmann's (Na 131, K 5, Cl 111, Ca 2, lactate 29), 0.9% saline (Na 150, Cl 150) and 5% dextrose (Na 0, Cl 0, calories 188 — equivalent to 50 g anhydrous dextrose) (concentrations in mmol/litre).

4. 0.9% Saline ("normal" saline) is not, in fact, a "normal" solution (one mole solute per litre of solvent): the excess of chloride in 0.9% saline may result in a hyperchloraemic acidosis.

5. Hartmann's (Ringer lactate) contains lactate as physiologi-cal buffer — this needs to be converted to bicarbonate in the liver. This process is impaired in a poorly perfused patient and the excess of lactate may contribute to the metabolic acidosis of shock.

6. A colloid is a solution containing fine particles (modern "plasma expanders" contain gelatins). Dextran, Haemaccel, Gelofusine and hetastarch are examples.

7. Hypovolaemic shock may be secondary to excessive diar-rhoea and vomiting or plasma loss in burns: blood is not required to replace this loss, just electrolyte solutions or colloid.

8. Blood pressure in a fit adult may not alter until over 25% of the blood volume has been lost. A rising pulse is a much more sensitive indicator of a reduced blood volume.

A tension pneumothorax

A. Produces tracheal deviation to the side of the lesion.
B. Is rapidly fatal.
C. Can be relieved with a needle in the second intercostal space.
D. Is diagnosed by mediastinal shift on the chest X-ray.
E. Is associated with marked subcutaneous emphysema.

FTTFT

1. A tension pneumothorax is life-threatening. There is no time for second thought — if it is suspected, TREAT IT and **do not** wait for X-ray confirmation.

2. The condition arises when a flap of lacerated lung opens on inspiration (allowing air into the pleural space), but closes on expiration (therefore acting as a one-way valve). The consequent rapid accumulation of air in the pleural space forces the mediastinum to the other side, additionally compromising the function of the non-injured lung.

3. Physical signs are increasing respiratory distress, cyanosis and tracheal deviation away from the side of the lesion. The pulse is rapid and weak, the blood pressure falls and neck veins are engorged. Breath sounds are absent and the percussion note is hyper-resonant. There can be considerable subcutaneous emphysema.

4. The immediate action is to place a large-bore cannula into the second intercostal space, mid-clavicular line, on the affected side. This will produce an immediate improvement. An elective chest drain (q.v.) will still be needed.

A chest drain

A. Requires an underwater seal.
B. Is ideally placed in the 4th intercostal space, mid-axillary line.
C. Is indicated in multiple rib fractures requiring positive pressure ventilation.
D. Is required for all pneumothoraces.
E. Size 16 Charrière is adequate to drain a haemothorax.

FTTFF

1. The main indications for a chest drain are
   - Pneumothorax
   - Haemothorax

2. A pneumothorax should be greater than one-third of the lung volume or causing distress; simple needle aspiration is an alternative (unless there is coexisting lung disease), or if very small it is left to resolve spontaneously.

3. An underwater seal is impractical in the pre-hospital setting: a Heimlich flutter valve or urine drainage bag with one-way valve is then suitable.

4. It should be assumed that a traumatic pneumothorax will be associated with some degree of haemothorax. A chest drain in the second intercostal space, mid-clavicular line (appropriate for a "spontaneous" pneumothorax), will not provide adequate drainage and, when siting the drain blind without X-ray confirmation (i.e. "in the field"), the 4th or 5th intercostal space, mid-axillary line, should be used. A more basal drain can always be inserted later.

5. Charrière is the French gauge denoting the size of the drainage tube. 16 Ch is very small and would not be adequate to drain a haemothorax — more appropriate size is 28–32 Ch.

6. Positive-pressure ventilation will force an existing pneumothorax under tension: prophylactic chest drains may be inserted to prevent the likelihood of this in the presence of multiple/bilateral rib fractures.

A traumatic cardiac tamponade

A. Is suspected when the heart sounds are muffled and neck veins collapsed.

B. Is a cause of electro-mechanical dissociation.

C. Requires a rapid intravenous fluid challenge.

D. Is unlikely to improve with aspiration of less than 250 ml of blood.

E. Should be suspected in a steering-wheel injury.

FTFFT

1. A traumatic cardiac tamponade is the result of a penetrating (e.g. knife) or blunt (e.g. steering-wheel) injury to the chest. Blood within the non-compliant pericardium splints the heart, preventing normal diastolic chamber filling, and leads to a fall in cardiac output (and subsequent reflex tachycardia).

2. Hypotension is evident, with a raised jugular venous pressure (JVP) and muffled heart sounds (*Beck's Triad*); there is a further rise in the JVP with inspiration (Kussmaul's sign). Pulsus paradoxus also occurs (fall in pulse volume on inspiration). If there is associated hypovolaemia, the neck veins may not be distended.

3. Treatment is with urgent needle paracentesis, not intravenous volume expansion. Removal of as little as 50 ml can produce a dramatic recovery.

4. The sub-xiphisternal route is the most commonly used, wtih the needle inserted between the xiphisternum and left costal margin at 30−45 degrees and directed towards the left shoulder. The left parasternal approach is an alternative (4th/5th intercostal space on the left), but is more likely to be complicated by pneumothorax, internal mammary artery or coronary artery laceration.

5. Needle paracentesis will be of little benefit if the blood has clotted and at best will only provide a temporary improvement: definitive surgery (thoracotomy and pericardotomy) should not be delayed.

Open-chest cardio-pulmonary resuscitation

A. Is indicated in traumatic cardiac tamponade.
B. Access is obtained by sternotomy.
C. Should be considered in intractable ventricular fibrillation secondary to hypothermia.
D. Provides greater perfusion pressures than closed chest compressions.
E. Is often complicated by infection.

TFTTF

1. Open-chest cardio-pulmonary resuscitation was widely used before closed-chest compressions gained popularity in the 1960s.

2. Perfusion pressures are substantially better than with closed-chest compressions and the brain can be supported for up to 1−2 hours.

3. The main indication is thoracic trauma:

   - To relieve a cardiac tamponade and suture the lacerated myocardium (e.g. in a stab wound)
   - To clamp persistently bleeding vessels in the chest

4. Other circumstances in which it is valuable are

   - To temporarily clamp the thoracic aorta above the diaphragm (in severe intra-abdominal haemorrhage)
   - To remove a large pulmonary embolus
   - To allow direct warming (with saline packs) and internal countershocks to a hypothermic heart in intractable fibrillation (energy requirements are much lower and in the order of 5−40 joules)
   - When closed-chest compressions are ineffectual (severe kyphosis or emphysema)

5. It is performed through a left-sided incision in the 4th/5th intercostal space. The ribs are held apart with a rib-spreader. Compressions are between thumb anteriorly and fingers posteriorly, or bimanually.

6. The patient must be intubated and lung inflation must be maintained during thoracotomy by continuous positive-pressure ventilation.

7. Infection is not an important complication.

In a patient with head injuries

A. Hypotension is readily explained by intracranial bleeding.
B. Dilating pupils are a late sign of rising intracranial pressure.
C. The head injury takes precedence over chest and abdominal injuries.
D. The commonest cause of death is intracranial bleeding.
E. Brain injury produces rapid, noisy breathing.

1. The commonest cause of death in head injured patients is RESPIRATORY OBSTRUCTION. This is particularly likely during the period of temporary unconsciousness that follows the injury (owing to impact to the reticular activating system).

2. The AIRWAY is always the first priority, but the head injury itself will take second place to chest or abdominal injuries (which are more likely to need surgery).

3. As a rule, a head injury will NOT produce hypotension (except pre-terminally) — a search *must* be made for an associated injury.

4. Rising intracranial pressure results in a deterioration in conscious level, a rising blood pressure and a falling pulse; dilated pupils are a LATE sign. Breathing is initially slow, but becomes fast and noisy (Cheyne—Stokes also occurs).

5. Frequent observations are intended to rapidly detect any CHANGE in conscious level — a deterioration is an indication for urgent neurosurgical intervention. "Comatose", "stuporose" and "semiconscious" are subjective terms: the Glasgow Coma Scale provides reproducible observations between different observers. The scale has a maximum score of 15 and points are awarded for

   - best MOTOR response
   - best VERBAL response
   - best OCULAR response

6. **Remember**, the first X-ray in a head-injured patient should be the CERVICAL SPINE.

In injuries to the cervical spine

A. Extension injuries are commonly unstable.
B. "Spinal shock" requires rapid volume replacement.
C. A soft collar provides adequate neck immobilization.
D. Compression fractures of C1 are usually fatal.
E. C5/6 is the most frequent site of a fracture dislocation.

1. The suspicion of cervical spine injury in accident victims should always be high, but especially so in the unconscious and in those with facial or head injuries. Be wary also of the calcaneal crush fracture (parachutist; fall from a ladder), where heel pain may act as a distraction from the more important vertebral crush fracture.

2. In the unconscious, suggestive features of cervical cord damage include loss of sweating; flaccid, areflexic limbs; diaphragmatic breathing and priapism.

3. Fracture dislocations are most common between C5/6 and C6/7, the most mobile part of the cervical spine. Look for tenderness, neck deformity, motor or sensory deficit and loss of sphincter control.

4. An "unstable" injury is one in which the posterior ligament complex has been disrupted (supraspinous and interspinous ligaments). This happens most consistently with flexion + rotation injuries (motorcycle accident; diving into a shallow pool). Pure extension tends to avulse a bone fragment from the anterior vertebral border, but the posterior ligament complex is intact. Flexion produces an anteriorly wedged vertebra.

5. "Spinal shock" is the profound fall in blood pressure *without* reflex tachycardia, due to the loss of sympathetic vasomotor and cardiac tone. The vagus is then unopposed and stimulation (from endotracheal suction or hypoxia) can precipitate bradycardia or even asystole. The heart will not respond to a fluid challenge and there is a real danger of fluid overload.

6. A soft collar is NOT adequate support for an injured spine (**soft collars are for soft-tissue injuries**); use a spinal board or Hines cervical splint, which additionally fix the forehead and chest — alternatively, improvise with sandbags.

7. Compression fractures of C1 will only produce neurological deficit in 50%. If the patient is conscious they will have severe occipital pain (pressure on greater occipital nerve) and will support their head in their hands.

Concerning facio-maxillary injuries

A. 15% also damage their cervical cord.
B. Unconscious patients are evacuated face down.
C. Objects impaled through the cheek should be removed.
D. CSF rhinorrhoea is common in fractures of the middle third of the face.
E. Le Fort fractures will obstruct the airway and require immediate cricothyrotomy.

FTTTF

1. The commonest maxillofacial injury is a fracture of the mandible, but these are rarely associated with enough soft-tissue swelling to compromise the airway.

2. 2% of facial injuries are associated with cervical cord damage, but suspicion of this and an underlying head injury should be high with severe facial trauma.

3. The middle third of the face is the area between the tops of the orbits and the upper jaw. Fractures of this area are eponymously termed "Le Fort" fractures (after René Le Fort, a Parisian surgeon who dropped stones on the faces of corpses in 1901) and divided into types I, II and III. The face is elongated and oedematous, with circumocular bruising ("dish" or "panda" face).

4. Le Fort fractures are comminuted (often over 50 fragments) and unstable, and the detached facial bones are free to slide downwards and backwards along the incline of the base of the skull: when the nose is also blocked (by clotted blood) the airway is completely compromised. Relief can easily be achieved by pulling the hard palate upwards with two fingers hooked behind the front teeth.

5. Le Fort types II and III involve the cribriform plate and CSF rhinorrhoea should be anticipated.

6. During evacuation, conscious patients may prefer to sit with their heads held forwards. The airway of unconscious patients is best protected by lying them face down with their head hanging over the end of the stretcher, and forehead supported between the stretcher poles by a bandage. This allows free drainage of blood, vomit and broken teeth which would otherwise be aspirated.

7. Blood loss from a penetrating cheek injury cannot be controlled until the penetrating object is removed. Direct pressure can then be applied to the outside and inside of the cheek simultaneously. This avoids further blood loss into the mouth, which places the airway at risk, and is probably the ONLY indication for removing an impaled foreign body.

In an adult who has fractured his pelvis in a road traffic accident

A. A high-riding prostate implies urethral transection.
B. And can not pass urine must be catheterised
C. Rupture of the diaphragm should be excluded.
D. Serum is grouped and saved.
E. Mortality is as high as 20% in cases of unstable crush injury.

TFTFT

1. Pelvic fractures result from direct violence or force trans-mitted through the femur. Isolated fractures (commonly of the superior or inferior pubic rami) are usually stable; fractures involving more than one part of the pelvic ring (as may occur with a road traffic accident, crush injury or fall from a height) are often unstable. Mortality overall is 5–20%.

2. The diagnosis is suggested by an inability to stand and pain on springing the pelvis. Bruising appears in the perineum, thigh and along the line of the inguinal ligament.

3. **Haemorrhage** is the most important immediate compli-cation — this can be severe and is likely to be concealed. It should be anticipated in all but the most minor fracture, but particularly when the pelvic ring is disrupted. Blood must be cross-matched immediately.

4. Rupture of the urethra occurs with a fracture near the symphysis, or with symphysial disruption, and is suspected when the prostate is high-riding and blood is present at the urethral meatus. If there is doubt, the casualty should first attempt to pass urine. A clear sample will rule out urethral injury. If no sample can be produced, or if it is blood-stained, a retrograde urethrogram will determine the site of the injury: do *NOT* attempt to insert a urethral catheter — this may complete a partial tear. Drain the bladder via a suprapubic catheter.

5. The bladder may be punctured anteriorly by a bone spicule, allowing urine to extravasate into the extraperitoneal space, or burst if compressed when full (usually at its dome or posterior surface), when urine enters the peritoneal cavity.

6. The rectum and vagina are uncommonly involved. Damage to nerves of the lumbosacral plexus (as occurs with dis-ruption through the sacro-iliac joint) is often permanent.

7. Remember to X-ray the chest to avoid missing the associated diaphragmatic rupture.

Following abdominal trauma

A. All penetrating wounds require laparotomy.
B. An imprint sign suggests serious injury.
C. Four quadrant tap is recommended.
D. Morphine should not be given at the roadside as it will mask abdominal signs.
E. Splenic rupture may be delayed for several days.

FTFTT

1. An "imprint" of clothing or rubber tyre mark will be seen on the abdominal skin when it has been forcibly compressed against the spine: it should arouse the suspicion of serious internal injury.

2. Splenic rupture accounts for about 50% of visceral injuries following closed abdominal trauma. One-quarter of these will be delayed for days (or even weeks). As well as shock, there will be peritonism and, after several hours, signs of ileus. Referred pain to the left shoulder is common (Kehr's sign) owing to diaphragmatic irritation by blood.

3. Morphine will certainly mask the signs of peritonism (tenderness and guarding) that a surgeon will seek before he considers laparotomy. This should not be a reason however to withold analgesia from a distressed patient who may need extricating from a vehicle before an uncomfortable journey to hospital. Under these circumstances, entonox is far superior as its effects wear off rapidly thus allowing more accurate clinical assessment.

4. Not all penetrating wounds require laparotomy — it is mandatory for a high-velocity injury, but stab wounds may not be associated with any visceral damage. In these cases, when the patient is stable, they are observed closely and examined regularly.

5. Four-quadrant tap with a needle and syringe is an unreliable method of detecting intra-abdominal bleeding, but if assessment of the abdomen is difficult (e.g. in the unconscious) peritoneal lavage — with a percutaneous catheter in the mid-line below the umbilicus — is worthwhile. The bladder MUST be emptied first and a nasogastric tube is advisable in trauma victims. Blood aspirated directly or after lavage with 1 litre of warm saline is a positive test (the open technique will avoid false positives from abdominal wall bleeding); pink-stained fluid (through which newsprint can be read) is generally not significant. Retroperitoneal bleeding can easily be missed.

Concerning a patient trapped in a car at a road accident

A. Morphine is a better analgesic than Entonox for combined chest and head injuries.
B. Injuries can be anticipated from the appearance of the car.
C. Impaling objects should be carefully removed.
D. Death is often from hypovolaemia.
E. Trapped limbs should be amputated to facilitate release.

FTFTF

1. The wreckage of a vehicle will give valuable clues to the injuries sustained ("reading the wreckage"): for example, a deformed steering wheel will suggest a chest injury, a side collision ipselateral limb and trunk injury, and a rear collision whiplash.

2. Other than airway obstruction, the common avoidable cause of death is hypovolaemia from blood loss. At least one large-bore cannula (14G/16G) is inserted and volume restored with colloid. If a prolonged entrapment is anticipated, blood can be cross-matched (q.v.) for transfusion at the road side.

3. Do **NOT** attempt to remove impaling objects (e.g. fence post or road sign), as uncontrollable blood loss may follow. The object should be carefully trimmed and firmly supported during transport. Beware of heat conduction to the patient through metal objects if they are cut thermally.

4. Morphine (q.v.) will depress respiration and interfere with neurological observation (by causing drowsiness and pupil constriction). It is *not* suitable for head and chest injuries. Entonox is a safe and effective analgesic in this situation, although patient co-operation is needed for the self-administration technique. Difficult, but painless, extrications of fractured limbs are possible if the patient is first saturated for several minutes with the gas.

5. Limbs are rarely so hopelessly trapped as to need amputation to facilitate release. If practical, two doctors should concur. Limbs discovered at the scene from traumatic amputation should accompany the casualty expeditiously to hospital (ideally in a clean plastic bag, kept cool with ice or instant cold packs).

A traumatic rupture of the diaphragm

A. Is more common with the right hemi-diaphragm.
B. Is a commonly missed injury.
C. Diagnosis may be helped by passing a nasogastric tube.
D. Causes respiratory embarrassment due to diaphragmatic palsy.
E. Is usually the result of a crushing abdominal injury.

FTTFT

1. A traumatic rupture of the diaphragm is usually the result of abdominal compression which bursts the diaphragm at its dome. Less commonly, the diaphragm is breached in a penetrating injury.
2. The left hemi-diaphragm is invariably involved.
3. In the acute phase it is often missed, but as herniated abdominal contents (stomach/transverse colon) start to dilate, respiratory embarrassment ensues, with cyanosis, hypotension and mediastinal shift.
4. Auscultation will reveal breath sounds replaced by bowel sounds and a chest X-ray will show the herniated abdominal contents: these may be variably misinterpreted as "acute gastric dilatation", an "elevated left hemi-diaphragm" or a "loculated haemopneumothorax".
5. A nasogastric tube can help in confirming the diagnosis if it is seen to lie above the expected level of the left hemi-diaphragm.
6. Treatment is early surgical repair.
7. The small tears caused by penetrating injuries (e.g. by knife) may have no attributable symptoms for weeks or months.

Traumatic aortic rupture

A. Is a common cause of sudden death after a road traffic accident.
B. Occurs at the level of the ligamentum arteriosum.
C. Can be confidently excluded by a normal chest X-ray.
D. Should be suspected when the first rib is fractured and trachea deviated to the right.
E. Results from rapid deceleration.

TTFTT

1. Acute traumatic aortic rupture is commonly the result of rapid deceleration, as occurs in a road traffic accident or a fall from a great height.

2. Sudden death is the usual outcome and only 20% will reach hospital alive. Death is particularly likely in the elderly whose aorta is rigid, whereas a partial tear might occur in a younger, more compliant vessel.

3. The most frequent site is the junction of the fixed and mobile portions of the aortic arch: this is at a level between the origin of the left subclavian artery and the ligamentum arteriosum.

4. Clinically it is suspected in deceleration or closed chest injuries with unexplained hypotension. A systolic murmur and blood pressure differential between the upper and lower limbs are described. There may, more importantly, be no specific signs and the diagnosis easily missed in a patient with multiple injuries and vague symptoms of chest pain and shortness of breath. A widened mediastinum on chest X-ray will only be present 50% of the time, but other X-ray features are also suggestive — these include an obliterated aortic knuckle, fracture of the 1st and 2nd ribs, deviation of the trachea to the right and depression of the left mainstem bronchus.

5. Aortography will confirm the diagnosis. Without urgent surgical repair the majority will die.

A posterior dislocation of the hip

A. Is suspected in a driver involved in a road accident who has a patellar laceration.
B. Produces a shortened and externally rotated limb.
C. Is associated with damage to the sciatic nerve.
D. Can be missed if there is a femoral shaft fracture.
E. Is less common than an anterior dislocation.

1. Posterior dislocation of the hip is much commoner than anterior dislocation (which is a very rare injury).

2. The mechanism is a considerable force applied along the length of the femur with the hip in flexion: this will occur when the knee of a car driver strikes the dashboard in the sudden deceleration of a collision.

3. Associated injuries are a fractured patella and fractured femur. A fragment of the posterior acetabular lip is often broken off and displaced posteriorly.

4. The limb will be visibly shortened, adducted and internally rotated (a shortened, externally rotated limb suggests fractured neck of femur); this diagnostic deformity may not be apparent if the femoral shaft is fractured.

5. The sciatic nerve lies behind the posterior wall of the acetabulum and is susceptible to injury producing numbness, paraesthesia and a loss of ankle dorsiflexion.

6. Anterior dislocations occur when force is transmitted through the femur in wide abduction.

In burns

A. The most important concern is the depth.
B. It is essential to know the time the patient was burned.
C. A hoarse voice suggests smoke inhalation.
D. Circumferential burns require escharotomy.
E. Considerable amounts of morphine are usually needed for full-thickness burns.

1. After the airway, the most important immediate concern is the extent of the burn, as this will determine the fluid replacement.

2. The extent of the burn is calculated using Wallace's "Rule of Nines", but this often results in an overestimation — a Lund and Browder chart is more accurate. Areas of erythema are ignored. The patient's palm can also be used to help estimation — it is roughly equivalent to 1% body surface area.

3. Infants have a relatively larger head, up to 14% of the body surface area, and their legs are relatively smaller (approximately 14%).

4. Fluid requirements are calculated from the TIME OF BURN and not the time of arrival at hospital: if there is a delay in starting i.v. fluids, half the total calculated volume must still be given in the first 12 hours post-burn.

5. Smoke inhalation is suggested by charred and sooted nasal hairs and mouth; hoarse voice and stridor are certain signs of laryngeal oedema and endotracheal intubation should not be delayed. Oxygen and nebulized salbutamol (2.5−5 mg) are given for wheezing.

6. Burns of the chest wall will impair chest expansion; around a limb, constriction will result in distal ischaemia. Relief is achieved by escharotomy along the length of the limb, or in the mid-axillary line/intercostal spaces.

7. Full-thickness burns are not painful. Anxiety is likely to be the greater problem and a parenteral benzodiazepine is more appropriate than morphine.

Fluid replacement in burns

A. Can be given orally.
B. Maximum requirements are in the second 12 hours.
C. Is best given as crystalloid.
D. Blood is replaced as 50 ml per 1% of deep burn.
E. Requires the weight of the patient for accurate calculation.

TFFTT

1. Intravenous fluid replacement is generally considered necessary with burns exceeding 15% body surface area in adults and 10% in children. Oral replacement is otherwise adequate, using a solution of NaCl and $NaHCO_3$ (Moyer's solution = 5 g NaCl + 4 g $NaHCO_3$ + 1 litre water, given as 50 ml/kg per 24 hours).

2. Fluid requirements are maximal in the first 12 hours. They can be calculated using the Muir and Barclay formula:

$$\text{Fluid volume (ml)} = \frac{\text{weight (kg)} \times \text{percentage burn}}{2}$$

This volume is given repeatedly over the following time periods (hours):

$$4 \quad 4 \quad 4 \quad 6 \quad 6 \quad 12$$

3. Other formulae (British Army formula; US Army formula) also take account of this differential requirement.

4. Hypovolaemia in burns is secondary to the loss of plasma. This is not only seen as weeping from the burn surface, but is also lost into surrounding tissues as a result of increased vascular permeability. The most important intervention is the starting of an infusion. In the United Kingdom, human plasma protein fraction (or human albumin solution) is used extensively, but it is **not** any better than crystalloid (as Hartmann's/Ringer lactate).

5. Blood is replaced as 50 ml per 1% deep burn, after initial volume replacement.

6. These formulae only provide estimations, and adjustments will need to be made according to the clinical response.

Concerning chemical burns

A. Acids are worse than alkalis.
B. Calcium gluconate is injected around hydrofluoric acid burns.
C. Burns from an alkali should immediately be neutralized with an acid.
D. Phosphorus burns should be protected with a dry dressing.
E. Chemical burns of the eye should be copiously irrigated.

1. Strong alkalis are usually more corrosive than acids.
2. FIRST remove contaminated clothing and irrigate copiously with water. This is particularly important when the eyes have been contaminated and should be continued for at least 20 minutes.
3. DO NOT try to neutralize the chemical (unless it is hydro-fluoric acid or phosphorus) as this will result in **heat**, which may further damage the tissues.
4. Any information about the chemical should accompany the patient to hospital.
5. Concentrations of hydrofluoric acid greater than 60% will immediately result in severe, painful burns. The antidote to these burns is calcium gluconate. This can be applied as a gel (2.5%) or dressings soaked in 10% solution. Persistent pain is an indication to inject the solution (painful in itself) subcutaneously around the burn: should this not be done, absorption of fluoride may precipitate hypocalcaemia and cardiac arrest.
6. Phosphorus is used in the manufacture of fireworks, ferti-lizers and insecticides/rodenticides. If it contacts the skin and is allowed to dry, it will spontaneously ignite and cause a deep burn. First aid should involve removing visible particles and covering the area with wet dressings. Phosphorus will react with copper sulphate solution to form phosphide, which is black and relatively inert. Copper sulphate itself can be absorbed, particularly if the tissues are breached and as such is highly toxic. It should therefore only be used under surgical conditions in an operating theatre once a general anaesthetic has been given and is used purely to identify phosphorus fragments, in order to facilitate their removal. It should not be used in any form of civilian pre-hospital treatment.

Electric shock

A. With an alternating current is more dangerous than direct current.
B. Fluid requirements exceed those expected from visible burns.
C. With high voltage is associated with long bone fractures.
D. Causes apnoea by paralysis of the respiratory centre.
E. From lightning produces death by ventricular fibrillation.

FTTTF

1. The first recorded accidental fatality from an electric appliance was in 1879.

2. Although alternating current can produce tetanic muscular contractions (thereby preventing the victim from letting go of the source), direct current will produce greater tissue damage and burns at the same voltage.

3. Entrance wounds are often very small and the degree of hypovolaemic shock, from loss of fluid into areas of tissue damage, will be out of proportion to the visible skin burns. Bone and dry skin offer high resistance, with low-resistance tissues (muscle and nerve) suffering greatest damage; moisture on the skin will lower its resistance, and may make the difference between a minor and fatal shock.

4. A high voltage across the brain produces loss of consciousness and apnoea; if respiration does not restart spontaneously, the heart will arrest in hypoxic asystole. A lightning charge across the heart (which may generate several million volts) will induce cardiac spasm: the heart will subsequently relax in sinus rhythm, but secondary asystole will ensue if associated apnoea is untreated.

5. Accidents with household voltage can cause ventricular fibrillation.

6. Long bone and vertebral fractures occur as a result of tetanic muscular contractions.

7. The priorities of treatment are to SWITCH OFF SOURCE and/or REMOVE PATIENT FROM CONTACT (remember to use insulating material); START BASIC LIFE SUPPORT (apnoea may be prolonged, but complete recovery possible); DEFIBRILLATION as required.

With injuries following an explosion

A. A high pressure is required to rupture the ear drums.
B. "Blast lung" manifestations are often delayed.
C. The majority of injuries are avulsions and traumatic amputations.
D. Sudden death may occur from coronary artery air embolism.
E. Flash burns are usually full thickness.

1. Explosions produce injuries from the blast wave, blast wind, thermal radiation, fragmentation and acceleration/deceleration. By far the most important are the injuries from missile fragments.

2. The blast wave is an "overpressure", travelling at supersonic speed. An overpressure of 30 kPa will rupture the ear drum, but much higher pressures are required to produce lung damage or abdominal visceral rupture; in the absence of ruptured ear drums, it is unlikely the patient has experienced a significant blast overpressure. With a particularly high overpressure air emboli are formed (perhaps due to air forced into damaged alveolar vessels) which may lodge in the coronary arteries (producing sudden death) or the brain (with neurological consequences).

3. The blast wind follows: this will disintegrate an individual close to the explosion. Further away it will avulse limbs and further away still will blow the patient over (acceleration injury) or against an obstacle (deceleration injury).

4. A brief pulse of thermal radiation will result in flash burns to those near the explosion — these are superficial, involving exposed skin (hands and face).

5. The majority of injuries are due to missile fragments, either primary (parts of bomb casing) or secondary (objects near to explosion); large fragments may also cause traumatic amputations.

6. The signs of "blast lung" may be delayed for several hours: suspicion should be high in anyone with ruptured ear drums. There may be no evidence of external injury.

With gunshot wounds

A. Low-velocity rounds produce a temporary cavity.
B. High-velocity rounds proudce damage distant from the track of the bullet.
C. All high-velocity wounds must be assumed to be contaminated.
D. The size of the exit wound is predictive of the degree of internal damage.
E. Gunshot wounds from a shotgun at 10 metres will produce severe internal injury.

1. The damage from a gunshot injury depends on the energy expended by the bullet: a small missile travelling at high velocity will be the most devastating. The density of the tissue and stability of the round will be important determinants in how much kinetic energy is exchanged.

2. Low-velocity rounds (travelling at less than the speed of sound, i.e. 350 m/sec) such as from a handgun will directly lacerate and crush tissues along the wound track.

3. High-velocity rounds (a modern military rifle will discharge a 3.6-g round at approaching 1000 m/sec) produce a pressure wave moving away from the wound track with a resultant temporary cavity. This cavity lasts only a few milliseconds, but is responsible for the severe tissue destruction often distant from the wound site.

4. Contamination is inevitable with a high-velocity wound: the bullet will carry a plug of clothing and skin through the tissues and further debris and clothing will be sucked into the temporary cavity.

5. The size of the external wound is no guide to the internal damage. A low-velocity irregular fragment will, because of its instability, produce a large wound, whereas a high-velocity ballistically stable round may produce small entrance and exit wounds, but cause considerable damage through cavitation.

6. A shotgun will cause extensive damage at short range (less than 3 metres). When fired from greater than 7 metres, pellets are unlikely to penetrate further than subcutaneous fat or deep fascia.

The "crush syndrome"

A. Could be expected to develop in a man whose foot was run over by a car.
B. Is a result of ischaemic muscle necrosis.
C. Will necessitate amputation if treatment is delayed.
D. Includes renal failure secondary to myoglobinuria.
E. Requires fluid restriction.

1. The crush syndrome will develop when a limb is trapped for a prolonged period (over an hour). A similar effect will occur with the prolonged application of a tourniquet.

2. The limb will swell, which will compound the ischaemia, and appear erythematous. There will be weakness, loss of sensation and severe pain.

3. Muscle necrosis releases myoglobin, which will block the renal tubules. Together with hypovolaemia from a loss of fluid into the dying tissue, this will provoke renal failure.

4. Tourniquets or compression bandages have been advocated as a first-aid measure to slow the release of myoglobin from the limb, but are not thought to be of any real benefit.

5. Treatment requires a vigorous diuresis of alkaline urine (which can be achieved by alternating 1.26% $NaHCO_3$ 500 ml, 5% dextrose 1 litre, and 0.9% NaCl 500 ml; frusemide is given to maintain the balance between output and input), which must be started within $2-3$ hours to be effective.

6. Amputation may be appropriate when presentation is late and the limb inviable.

7. When a car wheel runs over a pedestrian's foot there may not be any apparent initial damage — considerable soft tissue damage may later become obvious involving nerves, tendons and vessels, but this is not the "crush syndrome" *per se*.

The pneumatic anti-shock garment

A. Is contraindicated in pulmonary oedema.
B. Is suitable for stabilizing pelvic fractures.
C. Must be inflated to 100 mmHg.
D. Should be removed slowly, ensuring blood volume is replaced with fluids.
E. Works by auto-transfusion.

1. George Crile first used "external counterpressure", by means of a rubber suit, in 1903 to control hypotension during a surgical procedure in the sitting position. The idea of countering hypotension with a pressurized suit regained popularity after further development from the pilot's "G-suit" in Vietnam by Lt. Col. Kaplan: the Military Anti-Shock Trousers, MAST (or Pneumatic Anti-Shock Garment), were introduced in 1973.

2. The garment consists of nylon fibre wrap-around leg portions and a broad abdominal waist band, all secured with Velcro. Each portion can be individually inflated, but the abdominal section is NEVER inflated on its own.

3. Its main use is for restoration of blood pressure in traumatic hypovolaemic shock. The following mechanisms are believed to be important:

   - Auto-transfusion (750−1000 ml)
   - Increased peripheral resistance
   - Tamponade of bleeding points

   It is also effective for splintage of pelvic and lower limb fractures.

4. Pulmonary oedema is an absolute contraindication and cardiogenic shock a relative contraindication. It is considered safe in closed head injuries and thoracic trauma (despite the possibility of increasing local bleeding); theoretically the abdominal portion may splint the diaphragm, but in practice it does not significantly impair respiratory function.

5. The maximum inflation pressure is 100 mmHg, but the degree of inflation should be guided by the patient's blood pressure and NOT the pressure in the trousers.

6. Considerable caution should be employed during deflation, the abdominal section being deflated first. Adequate fluid volume replacement is imperative. Deflation is stopped if the blood pressure falls by 5 mmHg and further fluids are given until the pressure is restored. The garment may be left on until the patient is in the operating theatre.

Traction devices for a fractured femur

A. Reduce the mortality from this injury.
B. Reduce blood loss.
C. Are contraindicated with supra-condylar fractures.
D. Should be removed before X-ray.
E. May be applied painlessly after a femoral nerve block.

TTFFT

1. The first commercial traction splint was introduced by Hugh Owen Thomas in 1875 and bears his name — the "Thomas splint"; it is still in use in the armed services.

2. Extensive use of the Thomas splint in the First World War revealed that when used to immobilize a compound fracture of the femur, it reduced the mortality of this injury from 80% to 20%.

3. Traction is applied at the foot with counter-traction against the ischial tuberosity and surrounding soft tissues: in the case of the Thomas splint this is afforded by a complete, padded ischial ring. Other devices incorporate a partial ring (Hare/Trac-III) or padded bar between the legs (Sagar) and are generally simpler to apply. Both legs can be immobilized with a single Sagar splint.

4. The aims of a traction splint are to

    - Reduce pain
    - Reduce blood loss (this is largely a mechanical effect — the shape of an expanded thigh under traction will change from spherical to fusiform, which holds a lesser volume)
    - Prevent further damage to vital neurovascular structures
    - Prevent a closed injury becoming open

5. Traction should be applied with caution to supra-condylar femoral fractures: the distal fragment may be tilted posteriorly by gastrocnoemius and threaten the blood supply to the rest of the limb.

6. A femoral nerve block will produce anaesthesia (rather than just analgesia) of the whole femoral shaft periosteum, while additionally avoiding the systemic effects of a parenteral opiate (depressed consciousness and respiration).

Morphine

A. Is more readily reversed by naloxone than buprenorphine.
B. Is equipotent with diamorphine.
C. Has a beneficial venodilator effect in pulmonary oedema.
D. Is a schedule 2 controlled drug.
E. Is not recommended by the intramuscular route in trauma victims.

1. Morphine is an opiate analgesic, which acts as an agonist on endogenous mu and kappa receptors.
2. It is cheap and effective, but important side-effects include respiratory depression (dose related), hypotension and emesis.
3. Morphine should be given intravenously for relief of severe pain: give a 5-mg bolus followed by 2-mg aliquots. It should **NOT** be given intramuscularly to a shocked casualty, as poor perfusion results in poor absorption, which may prompt further doses — respiratory-depressing quantities will then enter the circulation on restoration of blood volume.
4. Diamorphine (heroin) has approximately twice the potency of morphine: doses should therefore be half those of morphine. It causes less nausea.
5. Opiate agonists can rapidly be reversed by naloxone (0.4−0.8 mg i.v.), but this often needs to be repeated as its half-life is less than morphine.
6. Buprenorphine (Temgesic) is a partial agonist and as such is less amenable to the effects of naloxone; doxapram may reverse profound respiratory depression in this case.
7. In pulmonary oedema morphine will not only allay anxiety and relieve any associated cardiac pain, but also reduce the pre-load by venodilatation and peripheral venous pooling.
8. Schedules 1−5 of "controlled drugs" represent the availability of the drugs to the prescriber (schedule 1 includes drugs such as cannabis and lysergide which are not used medicinally). Classes A,B and C represent the potential harm they may cause with misuse — morphine is in class A.

Entonox

A. Has a rapid onset and offset analgesic effect.
B. Is contraindicated in pneumothorax.
C. Can be safely given to a diver with shoulder and knee pains.
D. Is carried in black-and-white cylinders.
E. Separates at −6°C.

TTFFT

1. Entonox is 50% oxygen and 50% nitrous oxide.
2. It has a LOW lipid solubility — this ensures a rapid onset of action (because blood levels rapidly equilibrate with alveolar levels), but is responsible for its poor hypnotic effect (as it does not readily cross the blood–brain barrier).
3. It is a good analgesic, is cheap and non-irritant. It has no adverse effects on vital organs.
4. It is stored in blue cylinders with a white top (black with a white top contain oxygen).
5. Below −6°C it separates into oxygen and nitrous oxide, with the oxygen on top.
6. It can be used safely in head injuries, but only with great caution in pneumothorax as this may be expanded. It is ABSOLUTELY contraindicated in Caisson disease (q.v.).

Ketamine

A. Produces a tolerance state of dissociative anaesthesia.
B. Side-effects include sialorrhoea.
C. Causes profound respiratory depression.
D. Is unsafe in hypovolaemic shock.
E. Will allow phonation in adequate doses.

TTFFT

1. Ketamine (Ketalar) is a phencyclidine derivative used as an analgesic and anaesthetic.
2. Its action is to produce the state of "dissociative anaesthesia" in which there is profound analgesia, but only light sleep.
3. It has certain attractions for use in pre-hospital trauma because

    - Pharyngeal reflexes are not greatly depressed (*but* this does not guarantee airway protection)
    - It tends to INCREASE blood pressure, compared to most other anaesthetics, by increasing peripheral resistance *but* peripheral resistance is already maximal in a hypovolaemic patient)
    - It has a short half-life (intravenous effects last from 5 to 15 minutes and intramuscular effects from 1 to 2 hours)
    - It can be given intramuscularly (*but* absorption is unpredictable in the poorly perfused)
    - It can be used as a sole agent for analgesia and anaesthesia

4. Major side-effects include sialorrhoea and "emergence delirium" (vivid dreams, confusion and irrational behaviour), the latter being reduced by giving a benzodiazepine (midazolam 1−5 mg i.v. or 5−10 mg i.m.) at the same time — *but* this may produce the respiratory depressant effect you are trying to avoid.
5. Phonation and eye opening are normal with ketamine; involuntary twitching and limb movements are signs that more drug is required.
6. Ketamine 20−25 mg i.v. or 50−100 mg i.m. produce analgesia. 2 mg/kg i.v./8−10 mg/kg i.m. are suitable doses for anaesthesia.

With eye injuries

A. A saturated solution of glucose is used to irrigate lime burns.
B. Firm pressure is needed to control fluid loss from a lacerated globe.
C. A deformed pupil suggests a penetrating injury.
D. Patients should be evacuated on a stretcher with both eyes covered.
E. A fixed, dilated pupil implies an underlying head injury.

TFTTF

1. All chemical burns of the eyes need urgent, copious irrigation and tap water is acceptable as a first-aid measure. Efforts must be made to separate the eyelids, even if this is painful. Lime and other alkalis (e.g. ammonia) cause the worst injuries: particles of lime are difficult to remove (use a saturated solution of glucose) and are persistently corrosive.

2. If firm pressure is applied to a lacerated or ruptured eyeball, vitreous humor will be extruded with resulting blindness. The commonest site for a ruptured globe is the junction of the sclera and conjunctiva. These injuries can be missed if there is a preoccupation with a briskly bleeding lid laceration.

3. Penetrating injuries (knitting needle/dart) are suggested by a deformed pupil that reacts sluggishly to light; blunt ocular injury (squash ball/fist/champagne cork) can cause a "traumatic mydriasis" which may be permanent, and which could arouse unnecessary concern of an underlying head injury.

4. Casualties with eye injuries should be evacuated on a stretcher (to minimize movement and aggravation of the injury) at 30 degrees (intraocular pressure is lower than when recumbent).

5. If a foreign body is protruding from the eye:

    - **DO NOT** remove it.
    - **DO** support it (with a ring bandage/gauze squares).
    - **DO** cover **BOTH** eyes (conjugate eye movements also exacerbate the injury, including the bleeding from a damaged iris, which will be visible as a "hyphaema").

6. Amethocaine as a single application (0.5% eye drops) will anaesthetize the eye and allow examination. It should *not* be repeated routinely as it will cause corneal damage. Mydriatics (atropine 1%; cyclopentolate 0.5%) will often relieve pain.

Asystole

A. Survival is 10%.
B. Is the commonest primary fatal dysrhythmia in adults.
C. Is the usual cause of cardiac arrest in children.
D. In the absence of "P" waves requires pacing.
E. Should be treated first with atropine.

1. The commonest fatal dysrhythmia in adults is ventricular fibrillation; outside of hospitals asystole accounts for about 10% of cardiac arrests and electro-mechanical dissociation about 3% — the rest are ventricular fibrillation. The incidence amongst hospital inpatients of asystole and EMD is, however, significantly higher.

2. Asystole is the usual form of cardiac arrest secondary to hypoxia and childhood deaths are often hypoxic (i.e. primarily a respiratory death); it may complicate myocardial ischaemia as a primary dysrhythmia or secondary to other rhythm disorders (such as VF); it may also occur abruptly in conducting system disease (such as in a Stokes–Adams attack).

3. Adrenaline is given first, 1 mg i.v. Atropine is no longer considered the drug of first choice, but follows the adrenaline, and inclusion of isoprenaline in the protocol is no longer believed to be of any benefit (United Kingdom Resuscitation Council's 1989 recommendations).

4. Pacing is a last resort, but only if there is evidence of electrical activity (i.e. "P" waves).

5. **ALWAYS** check the leads and gain when confronted with a flat trace, and if possible change to another recording lead.

6. Survival from asystole or electro-mechanical dissociation is no more than 10%.

Electro-mechanical dissociation

A. Can be caused by hypovolaemia.
B. Is when mechanical heart activity is present, but dissociated from electrical activity.
C. Is a cardiac complication of tricyclic antidepressant overdose.
D. Requires cardiac tamponade to be excluded.
E. Is treated with calcium as the drug of first choice.

1. In electro-mechanical dissociation there is electrical activity in the heart (either normal or bizarre complexes), but no mechanical activity.

2. Mechanical causes should always be excluded. Look at the neck veins — if they are distended, consider cardiac tamponade and tension pneumothorax; if they are not, and the casualty is a victim of trauma, consider hypovolaemia. Other causes include pulmonary embolus and an overdose of tricyclic antidepressants.

3. Without any obvious mechanical cause prognosis is poor.

4. The recommended drug protocol for EMD is:

   (i) ADRENALINE 10 mls 1 : 10,000 i.v.
   (ii) Consider CALCIUM CHLORIDE 10 ml 10% i.v.

   Calcium could be expected to help when EMD is secondary to hyperkalaemia, hypocalcaemia or an overdose of calcium antagonists.

Ventricular fibrillation

A. Can be misdiagnosed as asystole.
B. Threshold is elevated by lignocaine and bretylium.
C. Has a worse prognosis than electro-mechanical dissociation.
D. Can be effectively treated by non-medical personnel.
E. Procainamide may work where lignocaine has failed.

1. There is no drug that alone can successfully convert ventricular fibrillation to sinus rhythm: the only treatment is DC cardioversion.

2. ALWAYS ensure that the gain is turned up on the monitor — you may otherwise treat ventricular fibrillation (VF) as "asystole" and the patient will certainly perish. If VF cannot be excluded, cardiovert three times (200 J, 200 J, 400 J) before starting the asystole protocol.

3. Lignocaine and bretylium will raise the threshold for ventricular fibrillation and facilitate cardioversion.

4. Procainamide is a Class 1A antidysrhythmic. Like lignocaine (Class 1B) it is a sodium channel blocker, but there is a prolongation of refractoriness (compared to a shortening). This difference is believed to explain why procainamide may work where lignocaine has failed, and vice versa.

5. The success rate of termination of ventricular fibrillation is upwards of 70%.

6. Automatic defibrillators will sense VF and discharge 200 joules within 60 seconds. Their potential lies with medical and lay (e.g. police) personnel not formally trained to use a manual defibrillator.

DC cardioversion

A. Is the treatment of choice for atrial flutter.
B. Of ventricular fibrillation requires synchronization.
C. Will result in a temporary failure of the defibrillator oscilloscope.
D. Delivers 160 joules to the patient when the defibrillator is charged to 200 joules.
E. Higher energies are used if the patient is digitalized.

TFTTF

1. Claude Beck in 1947 was the first to successfully use an electric shock to terminate ventricular fibrillation (VF), but it was not until the 1960s that it was used regularly in closed-chest resuscitation.

2. DC cardioversion produces a temporary depolarization of all cardiac muscle fibres (except those that are entirely refractory). It may not be necessary to depolarize all the muscle in order to restore sinus rhythm ("critical mass" theory).

3. The energy from a defibrillator (in joules, or watt-seconds) is displayed either as energy stored (in multiples of one hundred) or energy delivered (multiples of eighty), indicating there is some loss of energy between the defibrillator and patient.

4. The synchronization mode is used to avoid delivering a shock during repolarization ("T" wave), which can induce ventricular fibrillation. It is employed during cardioversion of supraventricular tachydysrhythmias when the "R" wave is sensed and the shock delivered well before the "T" wave. In VF no "R" wave would be sensed and the defibrillator would not discharge.

5. The oscilloscope takes 8–10 seconds to "recover" after discharging, during which time the monitor will display apparent asystole.

6. Cardioversion is the treatment of choice for a patient who is hypotensive and confused with atrial flutter. If they are taking digoxin, the starting energy must be very low (25 joules) as there is a risk of precipitating ventricular dysrhythmias.

Successful defibrillation

A. Is dependent on paddle pressure.
B. Is improved by antero-posterior placement of the paddles.
C. Is less likely immediately after another counter-shock.
D. May be enhanced by adrenaline.
E. Requires an adequate conducting medium between the skin and paddles.

TTFTT

Successful defibrillation is dependent upon:

1. The environment of the myocardium: hypoxia, acidosis, electrolyte disturbance, hypothermia and drug toxicity will all reduce the success of defibrillation.

2. The trans-thoracic impedence. This is the resistance of the chest wall. It is estimated at 50 ohms (range 15−150), but will vary with:

    (a) *Paddle pressure* − firm pressure (10 kg) is required

    (b) *Paddle placement* − antero-posterior positioning will reduce the resistance

    (c) *Paddle size* − 13 cm in adults, 8 cm in children and 4.5 cm in infants are optimal

    (d) *Paddle/skin interface* − use gel or electrode pads (gel is more efficient, but will spread with chest compressions and when heated by the current: this will lead to arcing across the skin)

    (e) *Energy delivered*

    (f) *Successive counter-shocks* − impedence is reduced: this explains why a second shock of 200 joules may be successful in ventricular fibrillation before the charge need be increased

3. The duration of fibrillation.

In myocardial infarction

A. The first ECG is negative in 5%.
B. Thrombolytic agents are contraindicated over age 65.
C. Over 50% of acute deaths occur in the first hour.
D. The left coronary artery is involved twice as often as the right.
E. Inferior infarction is often associated with bradycardia and heart block.

FFTTT

1. There are approximately 450,000 myocardial infarctions each year in the United Kingdom — 180,000 of these patients will die. The incidence is estimated at 6.2/1000 in middle-aged men.

2. Of those deaths that occur in the first month, over 50% will die in the first hour and most of these in ventricular fibrillation.

3. The left coronary artery is involved twice as often as the right coronary artery, but multiple vessel disease is the rule (triple vessel disease in 54%; double vessel disease in 28%; single vessel disease in 14%).

4. Inferior infarction is often associated with parasympathetic overactivity (bradycardia, hypotension, heart block) whereas anterior infarction is associated with sympathetic overactivity (tachycardia, hypertension).

5. The first ECG gives an obvious diagnosis of infarct in only 50%; 25% will be suspicious and 25% apparently normal.

6. There are few absolute contraindications to the use of thrombolytic agents, which significantly reduce the mortality from acute myocardial infarction. Listed contraindications include surgery within 10 days, cerebrovascular accident and severe hypertension; they should be used with caution after cardiopulmonary resuscitation. Given as soon as possible after infarction, they will aid recanalization. Streptokinase is the cheapest, but induces antibodies which inactivate the drug when given for a subsequent infarct (certainly if within the next 6 months) — recombinant tissue plasminogen activator (rtPA) would be suitable in this case. Anysolated plasminogen streptokinase activator (APSAC) is less antigenic than streptokinase and is an alternative first-line drug (especially out of hospital, as it is a single injection over 5 minutes).

Adrenaline

A. Will make a fibrillating heart more resuscitatable.
B. May be given down the endotracheal tube in half the intravenous dose.
C. Will dilate the coronary arteries.
D. Will enhance spontaneous activity in asystole.
E. Is inactivated if given with bicarbonate.

1. The goddess *Atropos* cut the mythological thread of life that was spun by her sister Clotho and measured by her sister Lachesis. Each thread was a man's destiny. Linné named the deadly nightshade shrub "atropa" because of its traditional use as a poison (the full name, "Atropa belladonna", also refers to the use of dilating eye drops for vanity).

2. Atropine blocks the effect of acetylcholine at postganglionic parasympathetic (i.e. "MUSCARINIC") receptors: these are situated on smooth muscle, cardiac muscle and glands.

3. Overdose abolishes sweating and leads to a hot, dry skin; pupils are dilated and accommodation is impaired; CNS stimulation produces anxiety and hallucinations. Treatment involves cooling and sedating (diazepam) with physostigmine (1 mg i.v./i.m. slowly) being the specific antidote (but beware of convulsions, bradycardia and bronchoconstriction).

4. Atropine will increase A-V conduction and heart rate and is useful for the symptomatic bradycardia or heart block (second degree — Wenkebach, or while preparing to pace Mobitz type 2) following an acute myocardial infarction. 0.6 mg is given every 5 minutes until the heart rate exceeds 60 per minute or a total dose of 2.4 mg administered. The tachycardia atropine induces is not necessarily entirely beneficial, as it will increase myocardial oxygen demand.

5. The effect of acetylcholine at NICOTINIC receptors (sympathetic and parasympathetic ganglia; voluntary motor nerves) is *not* reversed by atropine. The skeletal muscle twitching and paralysis that occurs with anticholinesterase (organophosphate) poisoning will not, therefore, be improved by atropine and requires an oxime. Atropine in doses of $1.2-2$ mg i.v. every 10 minutes will, however, be needed to control the secretions and ease the laboured breathing: with these improvements the dose can be reduced and dose interval increased, but prolonged treatment (days) is often necessary.

Lignocaine

A. Is started at 4 mg/minute after reversion of ventricular fibrillation.
B. Will increase the force of cardiac contractions.
C. Causes transient numbness and confusion after intravenous bolus.
D. Has been used by ambulance personnel successfully to reduce infarct mortality.
E. Has a half-life of 5 minutes.

TFTTT

1. Adrenaline is the primary drug recommended for use in all types of cardiac arrest (ventricular fibrillation; asystole; electro-mechanical dissociation). It is an α- and β-adrenoceptor agonist, but it is predominantly its α effects that are beneficial in cardiac resuscitation.

2. It is given as 1 mg i.v. (10 ml 1 : 10,000) or *double* this dose down the endotracheal tube.

3. At the cardiac arrest, adrenaline will make the heart more resuscitatable: peripheral vascular resistance and cardiac filling are increased with a subsequent rise in perfusion pressure to the brain and myocardium during chest compressions; coronary and cerebral vessels are *not* constricted — in fact, there is coronary artery dilatation.

4. Adrenaline will also stimulate spontaneous contractions in asystole (by increasing automaticity) and restore cardiac output in electro-mechanical dissociation (by improving myocardial contractility). Fine ventricular fibrillation is coarsened, making it more susceptible to counter-shock.

5. Bicarbonate may inactivate catecholamines given concomitantly through the same intravenous line.

Atropine

A. Will decrease atrioventricular conduction.
B. Acts at muscarinic and nicotinic receptors.
C. Poisoning produces hyperpyrexia and central excitation.
D. Overdose is treated with physostigmine.
E. Will be required in large doses in organophosphate poisoning.

TFTFF

1. Lignocaine is a Class 1B (Vaughan Williams classification) antidysrhythmic drug. Class 1 agents are sodium channel blockers: the rapid influx of sodium ions, which results in depolarization of the muscle fibre, is therefore reduced with a negatively inotropic effect on the heart.

2. This "membrane stabilizing" effect will, more importantly, increase the threshold for ventricular fibrillation (VF) and make the heart more susceptible to successful cardioversion. Lignocaine alone can convert ventricular tachycardia (VT) back to sinus rhythm.

3. A lignocaine infusion is started after reversion of VF or VT:

   - 4 mg/minute for ½ hour THEN
   - 2 mg/minute for 1 hour THEN
   - 1 mg/minute for 24 hours

   Some consider an infusion is also warranted (although it is not uniformly accepted) in the presence of "malignant" ventricular ectopics. These are ectopics which

   - Occur frequently or in succession
   - Fall on the "T" wave of the preceeding complex ("R" on "T")
   - Are multifocal (different complex shapes)

   They may herald VT or VF, but their presence or absence does not accurately predict the development of these dysrhythmias.

4. When given as a bolus (1−2 mg/kg) intravenously, lignocaine can cause a fall in blood pressure and deterioration in consciousness — cardioversion should then be performed immediately. Transient numbness, muscle twitching and convulsions also occur.

5. The half-life is approximately 90 minutes.

6. An intramuscular injection of lignocaine by ambulancemen has **not** been shown to reduce myocardial infarct mortality. Survival is, however, improved by fourfold when ambulance personnel/paramedics are trained in the use of a defibrillator.

Sodium bicarbonate

A. An 8.4% solution contains 1 mmol/ml.
B. May worsen the intracellular acidosis.
C. Should not be given concomitantly with calcium chloride.
D. In excess will produce intractable dysrhythmias.
E. Required dose can be calculated if the base deficit is known.

1. 8.4% Sodium bicarbonate solution contains 1 mmol/ml — which is why it is prepared in this concentration.

2. It is an alkali which is used to reverse the metabolic acidosis of cardiac arrest: however, it must be used with caution as adverse effects may outweigh potential benefits. These may include

   - Worsening of the acidosis if excess carbon dioxide is not first removed by hyperventilation (added bicarbonate will increase intracellular CO_2, which in turn will increase intracellular acidosis). Priority should be given to adequate ventilation rather than bicarbonate infusion.
   - Right shift of the haemoglobin–oxygen dissociation curve: oxygen is released LESS readily to the already hypoxic tissues.
   - Alkalosis — with its own malignant dysrhythmias.
   - Inactivation of concomitant catecholamines (adrenaline, noradrenaline, isoprenaline).
   - Sodium and osmotic load.

3. As a rule, therefore, bicarbonate is **NOT** recommended for routine use in cardiac arrest. It may be given after 10 minutes of arrest in a dose of 1 ml/kg (or simply 50 ml for an average adult). It is given in ventricular fibrillation after the 5th unsuccessful DC cardioversion.

4. Bicarbonate requirement can also be calculated by

   - Minutes of arrest $\times$ 0.1 $\times$ weight (kg)

   OR

   - Base deficit $\times$ 0.2 $\times$ weight (kg)

5. Calcium should not be given through the same intravenous line (as calcium carbonate is precipitated).

Calcium chloride

A. May be given down the endotracheal tube.
B. Should be given in asystole.
C. Is an inotrope.
D. Can induce a spastic heart.
E. Will potentiate digoxin toxicity.

FFTTT

1. Calcium is no longer recommended in cardiac arrest except as an inotrope in electro-mechanical dissociation secondary to hyperkalaemia, hypermagnesaemia, hypocalcaemia or an overdose of calcium antagonists.
2. It does increase myocardial contractility, but can induce a "spastic" heart (a prolonged contraction) and trigger coronary artery spasm.
3. Survival from ventricular fibrillation or asystole is not improved by calcium.
4. It cannot be given down the endotrachael tube.
5. The dose is 10 ml 10% calcium chloride.
6. 10−20 ml calcium gluconate i.v. slowly is effective in acute hypocalceamic tetany. Do NOT give intramuscularly as it is painful and causes tissue necrosis. If administered too quickly there is a burning pain in the arm and perioral paraesthesia, as well as its potential cardiac toxicity.

In a person who collapses unexpectedly in ventricular fibrillation ("sudden cardiac death")

A. 25% have no history of cardiac disease.

B. The majority can be shown to be a result of myocardial infarction.

C. Those who are successfully resuscitated have a high chance of recurrence.

D. Extensive coronary artery disease is usual.

E. Wolff–Parkinson–White syndrome can be the trigger to fatal ventricular dysrhythmias.

TFTTT

1. The "Seattle Heart Watch Study" (Cobb *et al.*) has provided information on the epidemiology of sudden cardiac death. It is defined as the sudden halt of effective myocardial contraction as a result of ventricular fibrillation (VF), ventricular tachycardia or asystole.

2. The majority of victims have extensive coronary artery disease (often triple vessel involvement), but only a small number of those resuscitated had ECG evidence of myocardial infarction. Up to 25% have no previous cardiac symptoms. It is suggested the primary VF is a result of temporary focal myocardial ischaemia in a heart otherwise "too good to die".

3. Those who are resuscitated have a high incidence of recurrence.

4. Trigger factors include cardiomyopathy and valvular heart disease (aortic stenosis), electrolyte imbalance (hypo or hyperkalaemia; hypercalcaemia) and Wolff—Parkinson—White syndrome; young adults have died suddenly while exercising.

5. By definition, the identification of high-risk individuals is not easy. Frequent, multifocal ventricular ectopics *may* be predictive in ischeamic heart disease and in the months following myocardial infarction.

6. Recurrent, life-threatening ventricular dysrhythmias can be suppressed by drugs, but these are by no means omnipotent. Automatic implantable cardiac defibrillators (which deliver up to 30 joules directly into the myocardium) are an increasingly available alternative.

With a broad complex tachycardia

A. Ventricular tachycardia can be easily distinguished from supraventricular tachycardia with aberrant conduction.
B. It is safest to treat as a supraventricular tachycardia.
C. "Capture" and "fusion" beats suggest ventricular tachycardia.
D. "Torsades de pointes" responds to procainamide or lignocaine.
E. Hypotension is an indication for immediate cardioversion.

1. Electrophysiological studies have shown that the majority of broad complex tachycardias are ventricular in origin.

2. It is not easy to confidently differentiate between vetricular tachycardia (VT) and supraventricular tachycardia (SVT) conducted with aberration on a rhythm strip, but there are some guidelines. VT is suggested by (a) preceeding ventricular ectopics (if you are fortunate to witness the onset of the dysrhythmia); (b) "capture" beats (an interspersed sinus beat) and "fusion" beats (a hybrid sinus and ventricular beat); (c) precordial concordance (deflections in V-leads are either all positive or all negative).

3. If there is doubt **TREAT AS VT**. A very small number of ventricular tachycardias respond to verapamil (the treatment of choice for SVT), but haemodynamic collapse is more likely.

4. "Torsades de pointes" is a variant of VT in which the axis constantly changes. Unlike standard VT, it may be *aggravated* by Class 1 antidysrhythmics and these should be avoided. A search should be made for underlying causes (hypokalaemia, hypomognesaemia, drug toxicity).

5. If the patient is conscious and well-perfused oxygen, analgesia and antidysrhythmic drugs are tried first. If a bolus of lignocaine 100 mg i.v. fails, give further lignocaine 0.5 mg/ every 5 minutes to a maximum of 300 mg *or* bretylium 5 mg/kg over 8−10 minutes *or* procainamide 100 mg every 5 minutes to a maximum of 1 g.

6. Hypotension and impaired consciousness are indications for sedation and cardioversion. VT is then treated along the same lines as VF.

A sinus bradycardia

A. Of below 50 beats per minute after an infarct must be treated with atropine.
B. Is common after an inferior myocardial infarct.
C. Is part of the "Cushing reflex" in rising intracranial pressure.
D. Accompanied by "J" waves on the ECG suggests hypothyroidism.
E. Resulting from vagal stimulation occurs with morphine.

FTTFT

1. Sinus bradycardia is a heart rate below 60 beats per minute. It is a normal finding in a fit adult. It is also a feature of hypothyroidism, hypothermia, β-blocker overdose and cholestatic jaundice.

2. It is common after an inferior myocardial infarction. The absolute rate is less important than the state of perfusion (but this *will* often be unsatisfactory below 50 bpm). Treatment is with repeated doses of atropine to a maximum of 2.4 mg — if this fails to restore perfusion and increase the rate to above 60 bpm, a temporary pacemaker should be inserted.

3. "J" waves are an ECG characteristic of hypothermia (although hypothermia occurs with myxoedema coma).

4. With a rise in intracranial pressure, cerebral perfusion falls. To combat this systemic arterial pressure increases (but the pulse reflexly slows owing to baroreceptor stimulation). This is the "Cushing reflex".

5. One of morphine's cardiovascular effects is to stimulate the vagal centre with resultant bradycardia.

A subclavian line

A. Is the preferred route of fluid resuscitation in hypovolaemic shock.
B. Must be used to give the drugs in a cardiac arrest.
C. May be complicated by pneumothorax.
D. Is dangerous to insert in a sitting patient.
E. Directed too superiorly will enter the subclavian artery.

1. The subclavian vein is cannulated where it lies behind the medial third of the clavicle. It is separated from the subclavian artery posteriorly by scalenus anterior.

2. Important immediate complications of subclavian vein catheterization are pneumothorax, entering the subclavian artery, misplaced catheter (usually up into the internal jugular vein) and brachial plexus damage.

3. It is primarily a MONITORING line for central venous pressure measurements. Cold intravenous fluids given directly into the right heart can induce dysrhythmias. In an entrapment victim, however, a subclavian/internal jugular/external jugular line may have to be used for fluid resuscitation if standard peripheral sites are inaccessible.

4. The patient should be positioned head down (Trendelenburg position) while the catheter is inserted — this will prevent dangerous air embolism.

5. It is quite acceptable for drugs to be administered via a peripheral line (antecubital fossa) in a cardiac arrest — the arm is subsequently lifted (to utilize gravity) and fluids are flushed through the line. Theoretically a central line is attractive, but it is time-consuming and carries the above list of complications: it is not suitable for the pre-hospital management of a cardiac arrest.

In acute pulmonary oedema

A. Morphine is not given with a history of chronic respiratory disease.
B. Silent myocardial infarction should be excluded.
C. Early improvement after frusemide is due to a venodilator effect.
D. Aminophylline is added when diuretics have failed.
E. Venesection may be appropriate.

FTTTT

1. FIRST reassure the patient, sit them up and give oxygen.
2. Frusemide 40 mg i.v. will produce an improvement within a few minutes, owing to a venodilator effect, before any diuresis is apparent. If intravenous access is difficult, a crushed 40-mg tablet of frusemide sublingually will act within a few more minutes, and certainly more predictably than an intramuscular injection in a poorly perfused patient.
3. Morphine (or diamorphine) allays anxiety and reduces the cardiac preload, again by peripheral venodilatation. Its benefits will outweigh the potential risks of respiratory depression, even in the patient with chronic respiratory disease — in this group it would be wise, however, to start with a small dose. Naloxone should always be available.
4. Aminophylline may benefit when diuretics alone have failed. 5 mg/kg i.v. is the bolus dose, given slowly over 30 minutes with an infusion at 0.5 mg/kg per hr to follow.
5. Other venodilators (isosorbide dinitrate infusion) also have a role. Venesection is reserved for those who do not respond to the standard treatment: these patients may also need positive-pressure ventilation.
6. In the absence of drugs, rotating venous tourniquets are unlikely to be of any help.

In acute anaphylaxis

A. Noradrenaline is preferable to adrenaline.
B. Antihistamines are given.
C. Volume replacement may be necessary.
D. Steroids have an effect within 30 minutes.
E. The upper airway must be observed.

FTTFT

1. Acute anaphylaxis is a Type 1 allergic response which may commonly be precipitated by drugs (e.g. penicillin) and insect stings (wasp/bee).

2. Onset is usually less than 1 hour after the drug, but within minutes if given intravenously.

3. Noradrenaline has a strong α-adrenergic action (therefore maintaining the blood pressure by vasoconstriction), but no β-adrenergic effect (bronchodilatation): although adrenaline is a weaker α-agonist it *is* a β-agonist and is therefore used in preference to noradrenaline.

4. Adrenaline is given as 1 ml 1:1000 (i.e. 1 g) intramuscularly; subcutaneously it is poorly absorbed in the shocked state, and unless an intravenous dose is given very carefully it can precipitate ventricular fibrillation. It may be repeated after 3−5 minutes.

5. An H_1-antagonist (chlorpheniramine 10 mg i.v.) is appropriate as histamine is undoubtedly one of the mediators.

6. Steroids (100−200 mg hydrocortisone i.v. or 40−60 mg prednisolone orally) will have no effect for 30 minutes and their effect will not peak for several hours.

7. The upper airway must be carefully observed − obstruction may require emergency cricothyrotomy. Bronchoconstriction is treated in the same way as acute asthma.

In epilepsy

A. Witnessed convulsions should immediately receive intravenous diazepam.

B. "Status epilepticus" is repeated seizures without recovery for 1 hour.

C. Diazepam is effective intramuscularly and rectally.

D. Phenytoin given rapidly intravenously may precipitate heart block and hypotension.

E. A chlormethiazole infusion can cause respiratory depression.

FFFTT

1. Most grand mal seizures will stop spontaneously without the need for an anticonvulsant. A single convulsion (or repeated convulsions without recovery) lasting more than 10 minutes is termed "status epilepticus" and is a medical emergency: without treatment, permanent neuronal damage can occur after 20–30 minutes.

2. The priorities are to:

   - MAINTAIN THE AIRWAY
   - PREVENT FURTHER INJURY

   But

   - Do **NOT** force the mouth open and
   - Do **NOT** forcibly restrain

   DO remove false teeth if this can be done easily.
   DO place the casualty in the recovery position (to minimize the chance of aspiration).
   A nasopharyngeal airway is ideal and supplemental oxygen given through a face mask.

3. The drug of first choice is diazepam 10 mg i.v. statim and repeated after 5 minutes if required. This will be effective in 80–90% of cases. It is given as an emulsion (Diazemuls) which is less likely to produce irritant thrombophlebitis. The rectal route is an alternative, particularly in infants in whom i.v. access is difficult (paediatric dose is 0.3 mg/kg). Do **NOT** use intramuscularly — absorption is both unpredictable and slow. Fitting may recur within ½ an hour when the diazepam is redistributed.

4. If diazepam fails, use phenytoin. The dose is 10–15 mg/kg i.v. given at no more than 50 mg/minute (which will take 20 minutes in a 70-kg adult): any faster than this can precipitate cardiac dysrhythmias (heart block; ventricular fibrillation) and hypotension. Again, its absorption is unpredictable when given intramuscularly.

5. Chlormethiazole (Heminevrin) 0.8% infusion is an alternative to phenytoin: a bolus of 40–100 ml over 5–10 minutes will stop most convulsions. Titrate the infusion against the patient's response (usually 0.5–1 ml/min), but beware of respiratory depression.

6. Hypoxia, hypoglycaemia and hyperpyrexia ("febrile convulsion") are readily correctable reasons for continued cerebral irritation.

A 40-year-old diabetic collapses pale and sweating in the street

A. Hypoglycaemia is a likely cause.

B. Intramuscular glucagon may be given if intravenous access is impossible.

C. The cardiac rhythm should be monitored.

D. 50 ml of 5% dextrose will usually restore consciousness.

E. With a myocardial infarct the patient is more likely to die than a non-diabetic.

TTTFF

1. Hypoglycaemia is the commonest diabetic emergency. If early symptoms of a falling blood glucose are ignored (irritability, sweating, tachycardia) there is a danger of slipping into hypoglycaemic coma, with convulsions and irreversible brain damage.

2. Treatment of hypoglycaemia is oral glucose (2−4 sugar lumps/dextrose sweets) if the patient will co-operate, otherwise 50−100 ml 50% dextrose intravenously will rapidly restore consciousness. When intravenous access is difficult, 1 mg i.m. of glucagon will act within a few minutes. Glucagon mobilizes hepatic stores of glucose − if it is not given within 45 minutes of coma onset, these stores will have been mobilized anyway. On recovery of consciousness after glucagon, oral glucose **must** be given.

3. A complication of diabetes is autonomic neuropathy. Resulting postural hypotension is a cause of syncope, but more importantly the symptoms of hypoglycaemia and cardiac pain from an infarct can be masked.

4. Ischaemic heart disease is more common in diabetics, but they are no more likely to die than non-diabetics if they suffer an infarct. It would be important to monitor the cardiac rhythm − there may be a primary dysrnythmia causing collapse or dysrhythmia and injury pattern (S-T segment elevation) secondary to infarction.

5. It is unlikely that hypoglycaemic coma be confused with hyperglycaemic coma, as the latter will cause a gradual deterioration over several days, perhaps in the presence of intercurrent illness. If the patient is a known diabetic, is comatose and there is diagnostic doubt, **GIVE SUGAR**.

An asthmatic attack is likely to be severe if

A. The pulse is 90.
B. The peak flow is 100 litres/minute.
C. There is pulsus paradoxus of 5 mmHg.
D. No wheeze is heard in a distressed patient.
E. The $PaCO_2$ is greater than 5.3 kPa (40 mmHg).

FTFTT

1. Asthma provokes anxiety (in the doctor as well as the patient) which will lead to some degree of tachycardia: a pulse greater than 100 beats per minute is generally taken as an indicator of a severe attack.

2. Other indicators include

   - Peak expiratory flow rate of less than 120 litres/minute
   - Cyanosis
   - Pulsus paradoxus of greater than 10 mmHg
   - A normal or rising $PaCo_2$
   - A low PaO_2

3. A "silent chest" (that is, no wheeze in someone who is clearly having a severe attack) is an ominous sign: it implies that air exchange is minimal.

4. The normal range of $PaCO_2$ is 4.8–6.3 kPa. By hyperventilating, an asthmatic will reduce their $PaCO_2$ below 4.8 kPa. If this then starts to rise it indicates the asthmatic is tiring and requires ventilatory support: when it is greater than 5.3 kPa (40 mmHg) you have already delayed.

5. Pulsus paradoxus is a diminution of pulse volume in acute, severe asthma. A 5 mmHg difference is allowable, but over 10 mmHg is suggestive of a severe attack — in some cases it may be as diverse as 100 mmHg.

In the treatment of acute severe asthma

A. A β_2-agonist via a spacer is as effective as through a nebulizer.
B. A convulsion may be the first sign of aminophylline toxicity.
C. Air, and not oxygen, must be used to drive the nebulizer.
D. Diazepam is used to allay the patient's anxiety.
E. Ipratropium has an additive effect to salbutamol.

TTFFT

1. Strong, persistent reassurance will help alleviate anxiety: sedation must not be used.

2. Asthmatics suffering an acute attack are hypoxic and need supplemental oxygen — a nebulizer driven by oxygen should be used in preference to a portable air compressor.

3. Nebulized bronchodilators are the mainstay of treatment. β_2-Agonists (salbutamol, terbutaline) have an additive effect with ipratropium. Both are available as respirator solutions to be diluted before use with a nebulizer — hypotonic or hypertonic diluents should **NOT** be used as bronchoconstriction can be exacerbated. Single-dose ampoules (salbutamol and terbutaline 2.5 mg or 5 mg) are more convenient.

4. β_2-Agonists can also be effectively delivered through a spacer device, with which there is no significant difference between speed of onset and degree of bronchodilatation, compared with a nebulizer. Intravenously salbutamol is started at 5 µg/minute and increased to 20 µg/minute: this is at least as effective as inhaled salbutamol, but at the higher doses produces distressing tachycardia and hypokalaemia.

5. Aminophylline has a mixed acceptance amongst physicians. It must be given slowly (20–30 minutes is recommended, but over 5–10 minutes it is unlikely to produce toxicity in an adult) as an initial bolus, but this bolus should not be given if the patient is on oral xanthines. Toxicity results in nausea, vomiting, dysrhythmias and convulsions.

6. Treatment of an acute severe adult asthmatic is therefore:

   - Reassurance
   - Oxygen
   - Nebulized β_2-agonist 2.5–5 mg and ipratropium 250–500 µg
   - Aminophylline 250 mg (or 5 mg/kg) bolus followed by infusion at 0.5 mg/kg per hour
   - Steroids: hydrocortisone 200 mg i.v. 4 hourly and/or prednisolone 40–60 mg orally (then reduce)
   - Ventilate if exhausted or hypercapnic

In acute drug overdose

A. Ipecacuanha will give over 70% yield of tablets.
B. Gastric lavage must be carried out within 4 hours.
C. Activated charcoal is of most use with substances toxic in small amounts.
D. Corrosives are a contraindication to gastric lavage.
E. Salt water is a suitable emetic in the absence of ipecacuanha.

1. General measures in acute drug overdose are maintenance of the airway, support of the circulation and prevention of further absorption of the poison.

2. Promotion of emesis is more appropriate than gastric lavage in the pre-hospital situation. Syrup of ipecacuanha (which contains emetine) is effective in a few minutes. Adults are given 30 ml, children 15 ml and infants (over 6 months) 10 ml, followed by a glass of water in each case. The dose is repeated after 20 minutes if it does not induce vomiting. No more than 30% tablet yield can be expected.

3. **DO NOT** use salt water (which may cause fatal hyper-natraemia), mustard, copper sulphate or apomorphine as an emetic — they are all dangerous. **DO NOT** give ipecacuanha to patients with impaired consciousness — they are at risk of aspiration. **DO NOT** give activated charcoal at the same time as ipecacuanha — it will be adsorbed.

4. Activated charcoal (prepared from carbonized vegetable matter) will adsorb a wide variety of drugs and chemicals, but is most suitable for those compounds which produce toxic effects with low concentrations. 5−10 g is given, as a suspension, every quarter of an hour to a maximum of 50 g.

5. Gastric lavage should usually be performed within 4 hours of the overdose: exceptions are for drugs which delay gastric emptying (tricyclic antidepressants, aspirin). It is contraindicated after corrosive ingestion (oesophageal perforation possible) or with oil-based substances (aspiration produces a lipoid pneumonia).

6. Telephone numbers for 24-hour advice from one of the national poisons centres are displayed in the British National Formulary.

In salicylate poisoning

A. Children often present with metabolic acidosis.
B. Pulmonary oedema is an idiosynchratic reaction.
C. Coma is common.
D. Gastric lavage can be carried out up to 12 hours post-ingestion.
E. A forced alkaline diuresis is started with levels over 300 mg/litre (1.9 mmol/litre).

TTFTF

1. The lethal dose of salicylate is estimated at 0.2−0.5 g/kg (i.e. approximately 45−115 × 300-mg tablets in a 70-kg adult).

2. The patient will complain of vomiting, abdominal pain and tinnitus; they will be febrile, restless, flushed and sweating. Hyperventilation is a serious sign, but coma is unusual unless a massive overdose has been taken.

3. Metabolic changes are multiple. Stimulation of the respiratory centre leads to a respiratory alkalosis (the presenting feature of most adults) and the uncoupling of oxidative phosphorylation to a metabolic acidosis (the presenting feature of most children). In severe poisoning there is respiratory depression and carbon dioxide retention. Dehydration is common; hypo or hyperglycaemia and hypokalaemia are additional problems. Bleeding is a result of reduced prothrombin and impaired platelet adhesiveness.

4. Pulmonary oedema is an idiosyncratic reaction.

5. Tablets are removed by emesis or gastric lavage (effective up to 12 hours after ingestion owing to delayed gastric emptying).

6. Symptoms appear with blood levels greater than 300 mg/litre (1.9 mmol/litre) and significant toxicity with levels exceeding 500 mg/litre (3.1 mmol/litre). A forced alkaline diuresis is then started (or regardless of the blood level if the clinical condition is poor or if there is a history of more than 50 tablets ingested).

7. If the kidneys are functioning normally (the main route of excretion) half the salicylate will be excreted in the first 24 hours. The rate of excretion is increased by up to ten times with an alkaline diuresis.

8. A level of 1000 mg/litre (6.2 mmol/litre), or 700 mg/litre (4.3 mmol/litre) and rapidly rising, is an indication for charcoal haemoperfusion or haemodialysis.

In paracetamol overdose

A. 20 g is a lethal dose.
B. The patient is often comatose.
C. Therapeutic intervention must be started within 8 hours.
D. The antidote must be given intravenously.
E. Progress is monitored by the prothrombin time.

TFFFT

1. A lethal dose may be as little as 10–15 g.
2. Patients usually remain asymptomatic for the first 24 hours; coma during this period may be associated with other drugs (e.g. the opiate in a paracetamol/opiate combination tablet), hypoglycaemia or alcohol taken with the overdose.
3. Paracetamol causes liver failure through a toxic metabolite; this metabolite is usually inactivated (conjugated) by glutathione, but stores are rapidly depleted in paracetamol overdose.
4. Maximum liver damage occurs between 72 and 96 hours. Renal failure (due to acute tubular necrosis) will ensue in 25% with severe hepatic damage.
5. N-acetylcysteine will protect the liver by restoring gluta-thione levels — it is administered intravenously (150 mg/kg over 15 minutes, then 50 mg/kg over 4 hours, then 100 mg/kg over 16 hours); oral methionine 2.5 g every 4 hours to a total of 10 g is an alternative.
6. The protective effect is maximal when the antidote is started within 8 hours, but benefit will be gained up to 15 hours: after this time it may be associated with harmful effects.
7. 60% of patients whose plasma paracetamol concentration falls above a line between 200 mg/litre (1.32 mmol/litre) at 4 hours and 50 mg/litre (0.33 mmol/litre) at 12 hours are likely to sustain severe liver damage unless treatment is given.
8. Those with pre-existing liver disease or a high alcohol intake are at increased risk of hepatotoxicity.
9. Progress can be monitored with the prothrombin time; if it is normal at 48 hours, the patient is unlikely to come to harm.

In tricyclic antidepressant overdose

A. The pupils are constricted.
B. Sinus tachycardia is common.
C. Cardiac dysrhythmias carry a poor prognosis.
D. Physostigmine is given to reverse the anticholinergic effects.
E. Extensor plantars occur with mild poisoning.

FTFFT

1. Tricyclic antidepressants are commonly taken in overdose. Their pharmacology is complex, with important side-effects arising from their anticholinergic and Class 1 anti-dysrhythmic activities.

2. Symptoms of mild poisoning are brisk reflexes with extensor plantars, increased muscle tone, dilated pupils, sinus tachycardia, dry mouth and agitation. These will begin within an hour of ingestion.

3. More severe poisoning will produce coma, convulsions and cardiac dysrhythmias.

4. The majority will require no more than supportive care and measures to reduce the drug absorption. Most will recover within 24 hours.

5. Cardiac conduction abnormalities are common and the ECG will often show bizarre complexes. However, the tachycardia and dysrhythmias that occur with tricyclics do not carry the same prognosis as those following a myocardial infarct, are generally transient, and will not significantly impair cardiac function: antidysrhythmic drugs should be used with great caution (they may make matters worse) and are best avoided. A poor cardiac output is improved with volume replacement and inotropic support.

6. Physostigmine will reverse the confusion and coma, but only temporarily and at the risk of inducing convulsions and further abnormal cardiac rhythms.

The following are true in drug overdose

A. Paraquat is treated with Fuller's earth solution.
B. Iron may produce a fatal haematemesis.
C. Methanol is treated with ethanol.
D. *Amanita phalloides* (Death Cap) requires penicillin.
E. Atropine is given for the bradycardia of β-blockers.

TTTTF

1. Paraquat is an extremely toxic herbicide — a mouthful can kill, even if spat out. Erythema and ulceration of the fauces are followed by renal failure (tubular necrosis), the only route of excretion for paraquat, and subsequent accumulation in the lungs with pulmonary oedema. It may be detected in the urine colorimetrically. Treatment is with urgent gastric lavage (despite being a corrosive) and Fuller's earth, 250 ml 30% solution 4-hourly, which acts as an adsorbent.

2. An acute overdose of iron may result in haemorrhagic gastritis. Children are often the victims, attracted to their parent's coloured tablets (iron gluconate are dark red). Desferrioxamine is the antidote, given parenterally and down the lavage tube.

3. Antifreeze and paint-stripper contain methanol, which is converted by alcohol dehydrogenases into the toxic metabolites formaldehyde and formic acid. In the retina (where the enzymes are present for the conversion of retinol to retinene) damage is permanent with more than 10 ml. Death is possible with over 60 mls. Ethanol will inhibit methanol metabolism and is given orally or intravenously.

4. Ingestion of only part of one "Death Cap" mushroom (*Amanita phalloides*) can be fatal. Nausea and vomiting (*phallatoxins*) start after a few hours. Haematemesis, hypoglycaemia, liver and renal failure (*amatoxins*) are notable consequences. The principal amatoxin is strongly tissue bound: penicillin and sulphadimidine have been advocated to displace this toxin and allow renal excretion.

5. The bradycardia induced by β-blocker overdose does not respond to atropine (or isoprenaline): glucagon in large doses intravenously does, fortunately, appear to work.

With carbon monoxide poisoning

A. Symptoms include headache and confusion.
B. Hyperbaric oxygen is contraindicated in pregnancy.
C. Cellular respiration is inhibited (histocytic hypoxia).
D. Is commonly attempted using a gas oven.
E. The affinity for haemoglobin is ten times that of oxygen.

1. Carbon monoxide poisoning is produced by the incomplete combustion of carbonaceous material. Poisoning commonly occurs in house fires or can be deliberate (car exhaust gas is 3−7% carbon monoxide). It is no longer a constituent of household gas (methane).

2. The affinity of haemoglobin for carbon monoxide is around 210 times its affinity for oxygen. Hypoxia arises not only from the reduced carriage of oxygen but from a reduced release of oxygen to the tissues (shift of haemoglobin−oxygen dissociation curve to the left) and inhibition of cellular respiration (carbon monoxide combines with cytochrome P450).

3. The likelihood of toxicity depends on the concentration of the gas, the duration of exposure and degree of physical activity at the time. Early symptoms include headache, confusion and dizziness; coma, convulsions, dysrhythmias, papilloedema and pulmonary oedema supervene with more severe exposure.

4. The characteristic skin colour is "cherry red" (owing to the carboxyhaemoglobin), but pallor is probably more common and lividity occasionally occurs.

5. The treatment is

   - Remove from smoke environment
   - Start basic life support (expired air ventilation)
   - Give 100% oxygen

6. The half-life of carboxyhaemoglobin is about 5 hours — this is reduced to 80 minutes with 100% oxygen and further reduced to 20 minutes with oxygen at 2 atmospheres pressure (hyperbaric oxygen).
   Hyperbaric oxygen is considered for those who

   - Are unconscious
   - Have cardiac complications
   - Are pregnant
   - Have more than 40% carboxyhaemoglobin

In a child with suspected epiglottitis

A. There is often no history of upper respiratory tract infection.
B. The throat must not be inspected.
C. There will cyanosis and drooling.
D. Intubation must be performed immediately.
E. The onset of stridor is rapid.

TTTFT

1. Epiglottitis is a rare infection, usually due to *Haemophilus influenzae* (Pittman type b), in which principally the epiglottis is inflamed (and may swell to 10 times its normal size). The peak age group is $2-3$ years.

2. The onset of stridor (an inspiratory harsh sound) is rapid and without a history of upper respiratory tract infection. It can quickly progress to complete airway obstruction.

3. The child will be pyrexial, have difficulty in breathing and appear severely ill. Inability to swallow leads to drooling.

4. Under no circumstances should the throat be examined as this may precipitate respiratory obstruction.

5. Be prepared to establish an airway by cricothyrotomy, but all invasive procedures (i.v. access; taking rectal temperature) should wait until the child is hospitalized. Intubation should never be attempted without the facility for tracheostomy. Hold an oxygen mask close to the child's face while transporting to hospital.

6. Stridor is also caused by laryngotracheobronchitis ("croup"), a foreign body and angio-oedema.

In a Fireman who has been exposed to hydrogen cyanide (HCN)

A. There will be deep cyanosis.
B. The effects of HCN are reversed by oxygen.
C. Amyl nitrite is the preferred antidote.
D. Involuntary gasping occurs.
E. If exposed 30 minutes previously, he is given dicobalt edetate ("Kelocyanor").

FFFTF

1. Hydrogen cyanide is liberated when polyurethane foams and some synthetic plastics (e.g. PVC) burn. Along with its derivatives (acrylonitrile, thiocyanates, etc.) it is widely used in industry.

2. Cyanide reversibly combines with the haem component of cytochrome oxidase, thereby inhibiting cellular respiration ("histotoxic anoxia"). Acute exposure is followed by involuntary gasping after $15-20$ seconds and, depending on the dose, respiratory depression seconds to minutes later.

3. Blood oxygen concentration remains very high, since oxygen cannot be utilized by the tissues, and cyanosis does **not** occur until after respiratory arrest.

4. Oxygen is always given to those exposed to HCN as it appears to have a synergistic effect with the drugs given as antidotes. Alone it will not reverse the tissue hypoxia.

5. Thiosulphate is needed for the cyanide detoxification pathway in the body, but its action is relatively slow. Methaemoglobin will chelate the cyanide ion and up to 40% methaemoglobinaemia can be tolerated.

6. Sodium nitrite (10 ml 3% solution) is considerably more effective than amyl nitrite in forming methaemoglobin. Sodium thiosulphate (25 ml 50% solution) will convert the cyanide to inactive thiocyanate as it is slowly released from the methaemoglobin.

7. Despite this, dicobalt edetate (Kelocyanor) 300 mg i.v. is now the treatment of choice: cobalt chelates cyanide to form an inert complex. The dose is repeated after $1-5$ minutes if there is no recovery. It is highly toxic if given in the absence of cyanide poisoning.

8. The effects of HCN inhalation are very rapid, with death or inevitable recovery: prompt treatment may save the occasional life, but would not be appropriate 30 minutes after exposure.

Caisson disease

A. Is characterized by joint pains.
B. Should be suspected in any diver unwell after surfacing.
C. May involve the spinal cord.
D. Is a result of carbon dioxide bubbles in the blood.
E. Produces an urticarial rash.

1. A "caisson" (from the Old French "casson" and Latin "capsa", a box) is a large underwater chamber, open at the bottom (and kept empty of water by air under pressure) used for laying underwater foundations or repairing a damaged ship's hull.

2. Caisson disease (or "decompression sickness") is described in tunnel builders and divers. When air is breathed under pressure, nitrogen dissolves in the blood and tissues; this will be excreted by the lungs when the pressure is released — on ascent from the dive. If the ascent is too rapid, nitrogen will come out of solution as bubbles. This may manifest as:

   - The BENDS — joint pains (typically shoulders and knees)
   - The CREEPS — itching $+/-$ rash
   - The STAGGERS — brain and spinal cord symptoms
   - The CHOKES — shortness of breath

3. Any diver who feels **unwell at all** on ascent should be suspected to have decompression sickness.

4. Treatment is by rapid transport to a hyperbaric oxygen facility. The diving kit and the diver's partner should accompany the patient. Give 100% oxygen (to encourage the excretion gradient for nitrogen). Remember to use water in the endotracheal tube cuff/catheter balloon if these are inserted, otherwise they will deflate in the hyperbaric chamber.

5. Other problems associated with diving are

   - *Air embolism* — air trapped in the lungs (from inadequate exhalation) will expand on ascent, rupturing the lungs and causing (a) pneumothorax (b) mediastinal/surgical emphysema and (c) air emboli in the systemic circulation.
   - *The "narks"* — nitrogen narcosis, which produces euphoria and a decreased awareness of danger, but DISAPPEARS on ascent.
   - *CO_2 poisoning* — only likely in military divers who rebreathe their air (so that surface bubbles are not visible).
   - *O_2 poisoning* — will cause facial muscle twitching and visual disturbance, leading on to convulsions.
   - *CO poisoning* — rare, but possible when contaminated air (containing exhaust fumes) is compressed.

Hypothermia

A. Is when the body core temperature falls below 35°C.
B. Produces a consistent fall in cardiac output with temperature.
C. May induce atrial fibrillation.
D. Will cause death in 2−3 minutes in water at less than 5°C.
E. Is associated with hypertension on rewarming.

TFTFF

1. Hypothermia is a fall in body core (rectal) temperature below 35°C. In field conditions it may not be practical to measure rectal temperature, in which case urine temperature can be used.

2. Initially there is a rise in cardiac output secondary to vasoconstriction, but it will then progressively fall as a direct effect of the cold on the heart muscle and conducting tissue.

3. Below 35°C there is listlessness and confusion with possible atrial fibrillation; below 28°C ventricular fibrillation (VF) is likely and may be triggered by rough handling, rapid rewarming, a precordial thump, intubation or catecholamines (adrenaline/isoprenaline).

4. Temperatures below 24–26°C are incompatible with life — the cardiac output is insufficient to maintain even the reduced oxygen requirements in hypothermia.

5. It takes up to 15 minutes even in ice water for the body to be cooled — this time is shortened if the victim is young, has no clothing, is swimming or struggling or has little body fat.

6. If the body is rapidly rewarmed, "rewarming shock" will ensue: that is, sudden peripheral vasodilatation will cause the blood pressure to drop — it will also allow cold blood from the peripheries back to the core and precipitate a further fall in temperature ("after drop").

7. The treatment of a hypothermic individual can be summarized as:

   - AIRWAY (remembering intubation may induce VF)
   - SUPPLEMENTAL OXYGEN
   - SUPPORT CIRCULATION (cautiously, to avoid pulmonary oedema)
   - PREVENT FURTHER HEAT LOSS (remove wet clothes; wrap in foil blanket)
   - REWARM GENTLY
   - MONITOR (glucose, electrolytes, ECG, amylase, blood gases)

In casualties rescued from the water

A. Efforts should be made to drain water out of the lungs.
B. Death may occur rapidly after removal from the water.
C. Sea water is more dangerous than fresh water.
D. Resuscitation should be discontinued if there is no response at 30 minutes.
E. ARDS may develop in a conscious and ambulant individual.

FTFFT

1. Drowning is a common cause of accidental death. There is a high male preponderance ($30:1$ in age group $15-25$ years) and 20% of cases are associated with alcohol.

2. Twice as many drowning deaths occur in fresh water. This is **not** believed to be because of any important differences in physiological changes that sea water or fresh water may cause (namely haemolysis and hyperkalaemia), but is more a reflection of the opportunity to drown (i.e. one is less likely to be seen and saved).

3. The amount of fluid that is inhaled is usually very small (because of reflex laryngospasm), although a considerable amount may have been swallowed, which may be regurgitated during resuscitation. Time should not be wasted trying to drain the lungs of fluid as it is only delaying reoxygenation. In a small proportion, **no** fluid is inhaled ("dry drowning") — some of these may be sudden cardiac deaths on contact with the cold water, before any water can be inhaled.

4. Removal from the water may herald cardiovascular collapse: this is probably because the hydrostatic pressure of the water was acting as a pressure garment.

5. Prolonged resuscitation attempts are warranted, especially in the presence of hypothermia. Survival statistics are far better (70%) for those who are admitted with a palpable pulse ("near drowning") than those who are pulseless and apnoeic (8%).

6. All immersion victims should receive hospital attention, even if a "complete recovery" has been made. Respiratory distress may develop from 2 to 72 hours later.

7. Other factors to consider include:
    - Did anything precipitate the drowning (myocardial infarct; epilepsy; dysrhythmia)?
    - Is there an associated cervical spine injury (in a diving accident)?

8. In one form of drowning, there is uncontrolled inhalation of water due to a reflex tachypnoea produced by cold water on the face. This is believed to be the reason why many good swimmers suddenly drown in cold water. In addition to ARDS, frank pneumonia, often due to inhaled contaminated water may develop, as well as other infections, including leptospira when drowning has occurred in sewers or waters exposed to sewerage.

Triage

A. Means the sorting of casualties into three groups.
B. Is the "sifting" of casualties in order to determine priorities of treatment.
C. Priorities for evacuation may change after initial care.
D. Is performed once only.
E. Priorities will alter in the presence of mass casualties.

FTTFT

1. Triage is derived from the French word "trier", meaning to sift or sort out (but has nothing to do with the figure three).

2. The process was probably first used by Baron Dominique Jean Larrey (1766–1842), personal surgeon to Napoleon Bonaparte, who revolutionized the use of ambulances on the battlefield. It was certainly used in the Spanish Civil War (1936–39) to sort casualties into those requiring observation, operation or evacuation.

3. It is a *dynamic* process which may change at any stage of the evacuation chain: for example, a life-threatening tension pneumothorax will assume a lesser priority once a chest drain is *in situ*.

4. The system works as follows

PRIORITY ONE (critical)	Immediate life-saving treatment required, e.g. obstructed airway
PRIORITY TWO (serious)	Urgent treatment required, e.g. fractured femur
PRIORITY THREE (minor)	"Walking wounded", e.g. minor fractures/burns/ lacerations
EXPECTANT	Treatment deferred as the casualty not expected to live

DEAD

5. There are several casualty triage-tag systems: they have in common the ability to change the priority and space for casualty details. They may be colour coded (P1=RED; P2= YELLOW; P3=GREEN).

6. It is important to label a dead casualty "DEAD" to prevent a subsequent doctor wasting valuable time in repronouncing death.

7. In the presence of mass casualties the aim is "to do the most for the most": this will mean that those requiring difficult or time-consuming procedures will not be treated first, and it may appear that there is almost an inversion of the normal priorities. Some who are considered unsalvageable, but on whom at least an attempt at resuscitation would be made in normal clinical practice, will be left to die.

8. Triage may also be applied to the treatment priorities of an isolated casualty with multiple injuries.

Concerning resuscitation of the newborn

A. Cuffed endotracheal tubes should not be used.

B. Intubation is performed with an APGAR score less than 7.

C. Ventilation bags must be fitted with a 30-cm H_2O blow-off valve.

D. Respiratory stimulants (nikethamide/doxapram) are given for opiate-induced apnoea.

E. Acidosis is corrected immediately with 5–10 ml 4.2% sodium bicarbonate

TFTFF

1. As early as 1754 (Benjamin Pugh) mouth-to-mouth resuscitation was advocated for the apnoeic newborn.

2. After delivery of the head, the face and nose are wiped clean and gentle suction is applied to the oropharynx and nostrils (a strong stimulus to gasp). The baby is delivered into a warm towel and held slightly head down so that pharyngeal fluids can drain. Dry the baby and make a note of the time.

3. The APGAR score (**A**ppearance — colour; **P**ulse rate; **G**asping — respiratory efforts; **A**ctivity — muscle tone; **R**eflex response — to pharyngeal catheter) at 1 minute is a good indicator of the baby's condition, but calculating this score must not delay you from starting resuscitation if it appears immediately necessary (for a floppy, pale, lifeless baby).

4. A baby in good condition will have an initial APGAR of 7−10. With an APGAR of 4−7 the baby is blue and gasping, but the heart rate good: give oxygen by funnel for 30 seconds and if there is no improvement use a closely fitting mask and ventilate with a Cardiff (Penlon) bag. The bag should incorporate a blow-off safety valve (30 cm H_2O) to avoid over-inflation and pneumothorax. If there is still no improvement at 1 minute, intubate.

5. Cuffed endotracheal tubes are NOT used (to avoid tracheal damage) — a shouldered tube (Cole's tube) will reduce the likelihood of it being inserted too far and into the right main bronchus. Average sizes are 2.5−3.5 mm.

6. The baby with a APGAR of less than 3 will be immediately intubated and receive cardiac massage. Oxygen is insufflated via the "T"-piece arrangement.

7. There is no place for respiratory stimulants: in primary apnoea they are inappropriate (as virtually any stimulus will induce gasping) and in secondary apnoea they are dangerous (causing hypotension and convulsions). Opiate-induced respiratory depression is reversed with naloxone 0.02 mg/kg i.m.

8. Acidosis is corrected by ADEQUATE VENTILATION. If there are no spontaneous respirations after 2 minutes, 1 mmol/kg 8.4% sodium bicarbonate (diluted 50 : 50 in 10% dextrose) is given slowly via an umbilical vein catheter (5fg/8fg).

9. Beware of hypothermia. Use the Resuscitaire heater if available, otherwise ensure the baby is dry and wrap in a foil blanket ("silver swaddler").

10. The neonatal brain is more resilient to hypoxia (it has lower oxygen requirements; it can utilize glucose anaerobically), but resuscitation should be discontinued if there is no pulse after 10−20 minutes.

Concerning obstetric emergencies

A. Bleeding from a suspected placenta praevia is confirmed by vaginal examination.

B. The mother is placed in the knee-chest position with umbilical cord prolapse.

C. Concealed placental abruption is suspected in a shocked mother with a tender uterus.

D. A prolapsed cord must immediately be pushed back into the uterus.

E. Ergometrine is the only pre-hospital measure to stop an established primary post-partum haemorrhage.

1. Bleeding in pregnancy is classified as "early" (before the 28th week) or "late". Threatened and inevitable abortions will make up the majority of "early" cases of bleeding — this may be severe enough to require syntometrine (ergometrine 500 µg + Syntocinon 5 units as 1 ml i.m.) and an intravenous infusion prior to hospital admission.

2. All cases of "late" bleeding will need hospital admission and an absolute pre-hospital diagnosis is neither possible or necessary. If placenta praevia is suspected **NEVER** attempt a vaginal examination — to perforate the placenta with an examining finger would be disastrous.

3. Placental abruption ("accidental haemorrhage") is concealed or revealed. Bleeding can be considerable and can precipitate disseminated intravascular coagulation. A concealed haemorrhage is suspected if the mother is hypotensive and the uterus is tender; uterine rupture can produce a similar picture.

4. A prolapsed cord is an urgent indication to deliver the baby, usually by Caesarean. The mother is placed in the knee–chest position (kneels with her elbows on the bed or lies in lateral position with knees tucked into chest and pillows under her hip), reassured and given oxygen — Do NOT attempt to replace the umbilical cord in the uterus — handling it will induce further vessel spasm (already precipitated by the cold). Some would advocate replacing the cord in the vagina to keep warm and moist, but others do not handle it at all and cover with warm, wet packs. The presenting part should be held off the cord per vaginally until ready for delivery.

5. A primary post-partum haemorrhage is a blood loss in excess of 500 ml within 24 hours of delivery. It may result from uterine atony (largely prevented by Syntometrine with delivery of the anterior shoulder), a partly separated or partly retained placenta, genital tract tears or a clotting abnormality.

   ACTION: assess blood loss; establish intravenous infusion; massage the uterus and empty the bladder (may be preventing uterus from contracting into the pelvis); give ergometrine 0.5 mg i.v.; bimanual compression (one hand suprapubically, the other fist vaginally). It is probably not appropriate to attempt to remove the placenta (unless it is sitting in the os) until hospital is reached.

In a casualty who is bleeding profusely and who is HIV positive

A. The virus is absorbed through intact skin.
B. Betadine (povidone−iodine) will inactivate the virus in blood splashed on the skin.
C. The patient should not be attended by a pregnant nurse.
D. Needles should be broken or carefully re-sheathed.
E. It is advisable to wear a mask and eye protection

FTFFT

1. The human immunodeficiency virus (HIV) is largely spread sexually through infected blood, semen, cervical and vaginal fluids. It is also transmitted by transfusion of infected blood and blood products, by drug abusers sharing needles and transplacentally. It is NOT absorbed through intact skin (but may be through mucous membranes).

2. The virus is inactivated by Betadine (povidone–iodine 7.5% in a detergent base) which can be used to clean contaminated skin. Instruments boiled for 2–3 minutes or autoclaved are safe to re-use; work surfaces are wiped down with 1% sodium hypochlorite solution or alcohol.

3. Gloves and a plastic apron should ALWAYS be worn when handling infected body fluids. Latex gloves are thought to be superior to vinyl (but neither protect against needle-stick). With gross contamination, a mask and eye protection should additionally be worn.

4. **NEVER** re-sheath or break/bend a needle: if you do not stick yourself with the needle, you will at the least be producing a micro-aerosol.

5. Soiled clothing/linen is placed in a RED plastic bag inside a RED nylon bag.

6. Blood bottles must be clearly labelled "BIOHAZARD" or "RISK OF INFECTION" and the laboratory forewarned of their arrival.

7. HIV-positive individuals are invariably also excretors of cytomegalovirus (CMV), which can be harmful to the fetus. However, 50% of women of childbearing age have CMV antibody (implying persistent infection) and 40% of pre-school children will be shedding CMV over a 1-year period. The contact of pregnant women with the cytomegalovirus is therefore very common and pregnancy is *not* a contraindication to nursing a known CMV excretor (Advisory Committee on Dangerous Pathogens, 1986).

When managing the acutely disturbed aggressive patient

A. All should be physically restrained and receive a major tranquillizer.

B. Dystonia from haloperidol is reversed with procyclidine.

C. Haloperidol is effective orally.

D. A "bad trip" is treated with diazepam.

E. Amphetamine abuse is suggested by constricted pupils, bradycardia and hyporeflexia.

FTTTF

1. It is *not* always necessary to restrain a disturbed patient, but when it is necessary restraint alone can be sufficient to calm the patient without resorting to drugs. Clearly, major tranquillizers given in the pre-hospital/casualty setting may delay a definitive diagnosis and should be reserved, if practical, for use by the admitting psychiatrist.

2. If there is a risk of patients harming themselves or others, they should be restrained. Up to 5 people will be needed. Performed aggressively, restraint may only serve to heighten their delusions. Avoid pressing on the neck and chest — if they cannot breathe they will struggle more ferociously. Wrapping in a blanket can be very effective.

3. Haloperidol or chlorpromazine are suitable drugs. If patients can be persuaded to take the drug orally (haloperidol 10−20 mg), they will feel they are participating in their management. Haloperidol (5−10 mg) intramuscularly or intravenously will work more rapidly.

4. Dystonic reactions (involuntary muscle spasms — especially of face and jaw; oculogyric crisis) with phenothiazines/butyrophenones are reversed within a few minutes by procyclidine 5 mg i.v. or benztropine 1 mg i.v., but doses may need to be repeated.

5. Several drugs of abuse may cause (or unmask) an acute psychotic illness. Amphetamines ("speed", "uppers") produce a tachycardia, dilated pupils and hyper-reflexia with paranoia and hallucinations (tactile/visual/auditory); LSD ("acid", "blotter acid," "windowpane") produces a schizophreniform illness. Mescaline ("peyote"), MDA ("love drug", "ecstasy") and psilocybin ("magic mushrooms") are all similar to LSD, but less potent.

6. Mild, and sometimes severe, adverse reactions ("bad trips") will respond to strong reassurance and hand-holding ("talking the patient down"), but this is very time consuming. Sedation with diazepam or haloperidol is otherwise appropriate.

Concerning cold injury

A. Circulation of a frost-bitten extremity is encouraged by rubbing.
B. Small amounts of alcohol help to prevent cold injury.
C. A casualty should never walk on a frozen foot.
D. Rewarming should not be in front of an electric heater.
E. Frost nip will respond to local rewarming.

FFFTT

1. When exposed to temperatures below 0°C tissue will freeze. At first there are small, numb, white spots of skin ("frost nip") which respond to local rewarming (warm hand, warm breath). More extensive freezing is true "frost bite", when the skin is pale and waxy. Without urgent rewarming this will result in blistering and ultimately dry (i.e. non-infected) gangrene.

2. Alcohol is a vasodilator and will accelerate generalized hypothermia. When taken *with* exercise and *without* food hypoglycaemia will occur with as little as 30 ml of ethanol — confusion or unconsciousness will then further predispose to hypothermia.

3. **DO NOT** rub a frozen extremity — this will induce more tissue damage.

4. **DO NOT** reheat the extremity in front of an electric heater or other strong heat source — this may produce painless burns.

5. **DO** gently warm the extremity (with warm water bath at 44°C, or towels soaked in warm water).

6. **DO** protect against further general body loss of heat (sleeping bag/foil blanket or even polythene bag).

7. While a foot is frozen it is painless and can be walked upon. Once it has been warmed it is painful and any weight bearing will increase the tissue damage. If there are several casualties to rescue from a hillside, the frozen foot can safely walk.

Heat exhaustion

A. Is avoidable.
B. Is synonymous with heat stroke.
C. Is treated with cold intravenous fluids.
D. Occurs more rapidly in heat-acclimatized individuals.
E. Cooling is more effective with tepid water than with ice.

1. Heat exhaustion is fluid depletion through excess sweating. Heat stroke is a rise in body core temperature, which can occur with normal sweating in a hot, dry atmosphere but is particularly likely to occur if sweating is reduced (when sweat glands are inflamed — "prickly heat", "tropical anhydrosis") or the air is very humid (reduced evaporation); it also occurs when the temperature-regulatory centre is impaired (phenothiazines).

2. Heat exhaustion is often complicated by heat stroke.

3. Heat exhaustion is predictable and AVOIDABLE by increasing fluid intake. Those who are acclimatized to the heat are **more** at risk from heat exhaustion as they sweat more readily.

4. Treatment is with cold intravenous fluids — use 5% dextrose, since serum sodium and chloride are elevated as a result of haemoconcentration. The body surface is also cooled.

5. Tepid sponging allows continued surface heat loss through evaporation — ice will reduce the high skin blood flow and is a less effective method of cooling.

6. With heat stroke there is hyperventilation, confusion, a hot, dry skin and rectal temperature above 41°C. Pre-terminally the blood pressure falls, sweating ceases and the temperature rises even further. Treatment is **IMMEDIATE RAPID COOLING**.

When driving on public roads to an incident

A. Registered medical practitioners may use a blue beacon.

B. It is permissible to drive through a set of traffic lights at red.

C. You have right of way over other traffic.

D. The first consideration is to reach the incident as quickly as possible.

E. Headlamps should be switched to full beam during daylight.

FFFFF

1. The first consideration in driving to an incident is always SAFETY.

2. In order to be seen.

   - Medical practitioners registered with the General Medical Council are permitted to use a green flashing beacon fixed to the roof of their car ("Vehicle Lighting Regulations 1984", Part II, para II.2(1)).
   - Dipped headlights should be used.

   ### DO NOT

   - Use full beam
   - Flash headlights aggressively
   - Use additional fog-lamps
   - Use hazard warning lights while the vehicle is moving

3. In order to be heard.

   - The law at present does not extend the privilege of sirens or two-tone horns to doctors in general. However, in certain circumstances it may be considered that the vehicle is responding as an "ambulance", the doctor's skills and equipment having been specifically requested to the scene by the ambulance authority; this would also imply an exemption from speed limits.

4. It is a courtesy that other road users pull over to allow emergency vehicles to pass — you do **not** have right of way and a light/siren gives you no legal protection in the event of an accident.

5. Doctors should consider the following before driving to an incident in any manner other than as an ordinary road user

   (i) Are you adequately trained?
      - Have you read "Road Craft" (HMSO, ISBN 0 11 3407221)?
      - Have you received road craft instruction from a qualified police officer?

   (ii) Have you approached the local police to discuss
      - The use of additional illumination/siren?
      - The appearance (preferably white) and registration of your car (to be easily identified)?

In a helicopter

A. An intravenous infusion will speed up on ascent.
B. A "MAST" suit may dangerously deflate on descent.
C. Bleeding from fracture sites is aggravated.
D. Hypoxia is not a problem.
E. Divers may become symptomatic.

FTTFT

1. The advantages of helicopter transport of casualties are

   - Speed
   - Access (to difficult terrain)
   - Transport of skilled personnel and specialized equipment to the scene

2. The disadvantages of helicopter transport are

   - *General stress and noise*: reassure the patient and give them a headset.
   - *Vibration and turbulence*: may encourage bleeding and pain from fracture sites.
   - *Cold*: those who have been in the sea or on a mountainside are particularly at risk.
   - *Pressure changes*: the greatest pressure changes occur in the first few hundred feet. Avoid rapid altitude changes.
        ON ASCENT: an air-filled cavity will expand: pneumothorax, intestines (abdominal wounds may dehisce), MAST suit, endotracheal tube cuff, inflatable splint.
        ON DESCENT: infusions slow down; otitic barotrauma; MAST suit/ET tube cuff deflates.
   - *Hypoxia*: especially if anaemic; dangerous in the presence of cardiac or respiratory disease.
   - infusions slow down.
   - *Decompression sickness*: do **NOT** fly if you have dived 0–30 ft in the last 12 h or deeper than 30 ft in the last 24 hours.
   - *Aircraft limitations*:
        Suitable landing pad
        Weather conditions
        Flight checks (impose time delay)
        Number of casualties

The "HAZCHEM" warning sign contains information concerning

A. Methods for fighting a fire involving the chemical.
B. Personal protection required.
C. United Nations product number.
D. Suitability of the chemical to be washed down a drain.
E. The manufacturer.

TTTTT

1. Vehicles transporting dangerous chemicals must by law display an information panel with details about the load and how to deal with it should it be accidentally spilled.

2. The hazard is pictorially represented on the panel as CORROSIVE, FLAMMABLE (liquid/gas/solid), SPONTANEOUSLY COMBUSTIBLE, OXIDIZING AGENT or TOXIC. Mixed loads are shown as "!".

3. In addition, each chemical has an individual United Nations product number which will facilitate its rapid identification.

4. The "Hazchem Code" details how the hazard should be managed — what personal protection is required (and whether or not to use breathing apparatus); how to fight a fire (with water, foam, or "fog"); whether local evacuation is necessary and whether the chemical must be strictly contained or can be safely washed into the drains.

5. Further specialist advice can be obtained from the manufacturer, whose telephone number is also displayed.

6. The European system is similar ("KEMLER"), but only a hazard code and U.N. product number are included. A number repeated in the hazard code indicates an intensified hazard.

Concerning a casualty on a mountainside

A. Mild hypothermia will respond to inhaled heated air.
B. Morphine can be prescribed by non-medical personnel.
C. The police have responsibility for rescue.
D. Head injuries are the commonest cause of mountainside death in England.
E. Search-and-rescue dogs will trace the route of a victim.

TTTFF

1. The police hold the statutory obligation for mountain rescue, but they willingly surrender this responsibility to a Mountain Rescue Team.

2. The commonest cause of death on a mountainside in England is not trauma, but myocardial infarction.

3. Rescue of hillside or underground (caving) casualties will involve some time delay to mobilize the voluntary rescue team — critical patients will not, therefore, survive and intensive resuscitation efforts are unlikely to be necessary (as the victim will have reached a stable state).

4. Hypothermia is common and inhalation of humidified, heated air prevents further respiratory heat loss and produces at least a subjective improvement. Thermal ("space") blankets will insulate against body surface heat loss.

5. The unsupervised use of morphine by lay members of Mountain Rescue Teams has been allowed since the 1950s. Entonox is the alternative to an opiate, but is bulky to carry.

6. Search-and-rescue dogs (of the Search and Rescue Dog Association — SARDA) are requested at the discretion of the search team leader and are often deployed into the area before the rest of the team. They are trained to pick up airbone human scent (rather than follow a ground trail) and, if this leads them to a casualty, will return to and guide their handler.

In a nuclear plant worker who has received a large external dose of radiation

A. Will pose a radioactive hazard to you.
B. Diarrhoea and vomiting will occur within the first hour.
C. The prognosis of burns is worse than the surface area involved implies.
D. 450 rads (4.5 gray) is a lethal dose.
E. Death is likely within 12 hours.

FTTTF

1. Ionizing radiation (alpha-, beta-, gamma-, and X-rays and neutrons) emitted from a radiation source will induce cell nucleus damage in the victim, but the victim will *not* be a radiation hazard (unless they have ingested or are covered with radioactive material).

2. The LD_{50} (dose which causes death in 50%) in man is approximately 450 rads (4.5 gray). Survival is minimal above 600 rads, but probable below 200 rads. The elderly and very young are more susceptible to smaller doses of radiation.

3. Nausea, vomiting and diarrhoea will occur within an hour when exposed to the LD_{50}. With smaller doses than this there may be fatigue, weakness and loss of motivation. In both cases bone marrow failure will supervene in 2–4 weeks (but how early depends on the dose).

4. An exposure of 600–1000 rads produces intestinal damage and death in 1–3 weeks.

5. Supra-lethal doses can cause an early transient incapacitation and neurovascular damage (with cardiovascular collapse and loss of consciousness). Death is in within minutes or up to 12 days.

6. The prognosis of burns (thermal/beta- or gamma-radiation) is worse than that implied by the surface area involved.

7. Decontamination is required when the casualty has been covered with radioactive material (remove clothing and wash with detergent and water — this is 95% effective). In all cases of radiation exposure treatment consists of volume replacement, bone marrow support (platelet transfusion and granulocyte colony-stimulating factor), protection from infection and parenteral nutrition.

8. **Remember** RADIATION INJURY IS NOT ACUTELY LIFE-THREATENING — treat conventional injuries first.

Snake bites

A. Require antivenom routinely.
B. Should be sucked out immediately.
C. When a limb is involved a tourniquet should be applied.
D. Require antibiotics.
E. Bites from sea snakes are harmless.

FFFFF

1. There are three families of poisonous snakes — elapids (neurotoxic), vipers (vasculotoxic) and sea snakes (myotoxic).

2. Antivenom is only given if there is evidence of systemic poisoning, which may take several hours to develop. Early signs of envenoming are vomiting, hypotension and polymorph leucocytosis, as well as local swelling and pain. Immediate collapse is usually neurogenic (i.e. from fright).

3. Elapid bites may result in ptosis and respiratory paresis, sea snake bites in myalgia, myoglobinuria and hyperkalaemia, and viper bites in abnormal bleeding.

4. Incision and suction are not recommended — they will rarely produce any benefit, but will invariably lead to secondary infection.

5. The spread of venom in a bitten limb is reduced by im-mobilization. Firm pressure (in the form of an elastic bandage) is also helpful. An inflatable splint provides both of these.

6. If a tourniquet is used, it should be broad and lightly applied with only sufficient pressure as to obstruct lymphatic flow. It is unlikely that it would be applied correctly and is best avoided.

7. Antibiotics are not routinely required, but tetanus immunity should be confirmed.

Triage Exercises

Each exercise sets the scene of a disaster.

You are confronted with multiple casualties.

Answer the questions on how the scene is controlled and the order of casualty treatment and evacuation.
The letter against each casualty drawing is used to identify the casualty in the answer that follows.

CODE

P1 = **Immediate**   (life-threatening injury)
P2 = **Delayed**   (severe injury)
P3 = **Minor**   (minor injury)
Exp. = **(Expectant)**   (not expected to survive)
Dead

The Road Traffic Accident

A coach has crashed into an oncoming car on a country lane. There is considerable fuel spillage. You are passing in your car and stop to help.
There are the following casualties:

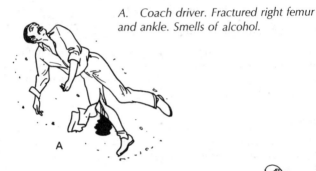

A. Coach driver. Fractured right femur and ankle. Smells of alcohol.

B. 70-year-old man. Central chest pain and shortness of breath.

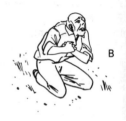

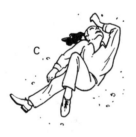

C. Glass fragment protruding from right eye.

D. 14-year-old girl. Anxious, short of breath, wheezing.

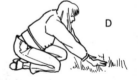

E.   Hit head on seat in collision. Was briefly unconscious: now feels sick and dizzy.

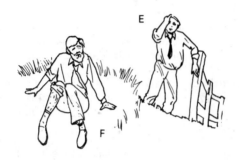

F.   Small wound on abdomen. Pulse 120. Blood pressure 90/50. Multiple other cuts.

G.   Unconscious. Slumped over steering wheel. Cyanosed. Noisy breathing. Right foot trapped by pedal.

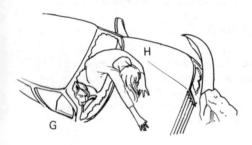

H.   Extensive head injuries. Pulseless. Apnoeic.

There are 12 other coach passengers apparently uninjured, but all tearful and distressed.

1. What immediate actions do you take?
2. What is your order of casualty treatment?
3. What is your order of casualty evacuation?

1. Immediate actions

SAFETY

- **Yourself** — Do not put yourself in unnecessary danger. Another casualty will help no-one. Wear a luminous tabard or coat to be seen and identified.
- **Casualties** — *Protect the scene*: park to protect the scene and use hazard warning lights plus additional illumination (beacon). Place a warning triangle.

    Prevent further danger: if in imminent danger (casualties lying in spilled fuel or in the road) then remove casualties immediately to safety.
- Turn off running engines and extinguish any other source of ignition.

TRIAGE

- Assess the number and severity of the casualties.

COMMUNICATIONS

- Take command.
- Collect uninjured/walking wounded together.
- Detail uninjured passengers to
    warn oncoming traffic of accident;
    get to telephone to alert emergency services;
    administer reassurance and first-aid under your direction to the injured;

2. Casualty treatment

1st   G   The driver of the car has an obstructed airway,
(P1) undoubtedly due to his tongue (this is the commonest cause of death in unconscious patients at a road traffic accident).

FIRST AID	**Advanced Life Support**
Extend airway with on-line traction to the cervical spine. Immobilize cervical spine before moving the patient.	Guedel airway and O_2 by mask *or* intubate (difficult in this seated position — a Brain laryngeal airway or pharyngotracheal lumen airway are

	Removing shoe may be all that is required to release trapped foot.	alternatives easier to insert).

2nd F
(**P1**) This man has sustained multiple cuts from broken glass. These alone are unlikely to produce this degree of hypovolaemic shock. He *does* have an abdominal wound and internal bleeding must be suspected (the superficial wound may be very deceptive in injuries from glass fragments).

Reassure. Lay supine or on side with legs tucked into abdomen (if position not already adopted by patient). Direct pressure and elevation to bleeding wounds.	Aggressive i.v. fluid resuscitation. Analgesia (morphine not contraindicated). MAST suit — if cannot stabilize with i.v. fluids.

3rd A
(**P2**)

Reassure. Direct pressure to wound. Splint one leg to the other, or improvise splint (e.g. wooden plank from axilla to ankle).	Intravenous infusion: titrate fluids against pulse and BP. Analgesia — gas (N_2O)/opiate (already has central depressant in form of alcohol)/femoral nerve block. Traction splint — this may be uncomfortable in the presence of the ankle fracture.

The consent of the driver must be obtained before taking a blood alcohol under the drinking and driving legislation, except under Scottish law.

4th B
(**P2**) This elderly man has ischaemic chest pain.

FIRST AID	**Advanced Life Support**
Reassure. Sit down. Give GTN if patient is carrying any.	Oxygen. Analgesia — if GTN fails and pain persists give i.v. opiate.

cont.

Monitor rhythm and treat appropriately.
Consider fibrinolytics:

- Aspirin 75—150 mg orally
- APSAC (available as single i.v. injection over 5 minutes).

5th	D (P2)	This young girl is having an asthmatic attack. Assess the severity (pulse > 100? Unable to speak? Cyanosed?).	
		Reassure. Sit up — may need to be in tripod position. Give β2-agonist inhaler if the patient is carrying one. Improvise spacer (e.g. with paper bag) if attack severe and give 10—20 puffs β2-agonist.	Oxygen. β2-agonist by nebulizer. IF β2-agonist FAILS - Add ipratropium nebulizer. - Consider β2-agonist infusion, aminophylline.
6th	C (P3)	Reassure. Do NOT remove fragment, but support with padding. Cover both eyes (eyes move conjugately and movement of unaffected eye may exacerbate injury). Evacuate on stretcher.	Analgesia/anxiolytic as required.
7th	E (P3)	Reassure. Sit down.	Will need skull X-ray and observation.
8th	H (Dead)	Pronounce this patient dead. Do not waste time in attempting to resuscitate, which could be used more valuably to help other casualties.	

3. Evacuation

If the airway of patient "G" is opened, his condition will greatly improve; the patient most likely to deteriorate is "F" and he should be evacuated first. Evacuation of other patients will depend on their response to treatment at the scene: for example, if it is suspected the elderly man has suffered a myocardial infarction then his priority for evacuation is high, but if his chest pain responds to GTN he will be one of the last to leave. A suggested order would be:
F G A B D C E H.

The Train Crash

A fast passenger train has collided with the rear of a slow-moving freight train and derailed. The accident is 10 miles from the nearest station in open countryside. You are in the rear compartment and are unhurt. The driver has been killed.

You find the following casualties in the front carriage:

A. *Fencing stake through abdomen. Pulse 130; blood pressure 95/55.*

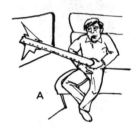

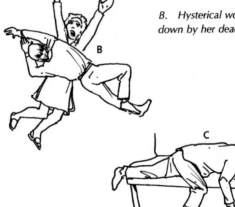

B. *Hysterical woman pinned down by her dead husband.*

C. *Extensive facial injuries. Difficult noisy breathing.*

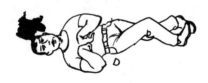

D. *Scalp laceration. Convulsing.*

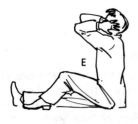

E. Hit on head by suitcase. Occipital pain. Supporting head in hands.

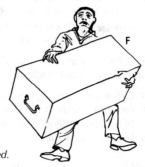

F. 13-year-old boy. Trapped by heavy trunk. Flail right chest. Cyanosed.

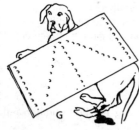

G. Whimpering dog, trapped underneath panelling. Open fracture rear leg.

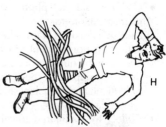

H. Legs trapped in twisted metal. Pulse 120; blood pressure 100/60. Foot pulses impalpable. Rigid abdomen, tender left upper quadrant.

1. What are your immediate actions (before observing casualties)?
2. In what order and how would you treat these casualties? (Consider the cases with and without other medical assistance.)
3. What is your order of evacuation?

191

10. Immediate Actions

SAFETY
There is danger to all passengers from:

- *Electrocution*: either from the "third rail" or overhead cables if they have been torn down. The third rail can be bypassed with a short-circuiting bar (carried on the train). The Guard will be able to advise on track safety.

(DO NOT assume the electricity has been turned off until confirmed by railway staff.)

- *Other trains*: the nearest signalman must be alerted.
- *Freight hazards*: is the freight toxic or inflammable?
- *Luminous clothing*/hard hat should be worn as soon as it becomes available.

TRIAGE

- Determine the number and severity of casualties (detail a member of each carriage to count the casualties).
- Do NOT get involved in individual casualty treatment at this stage.

COMMUNICATIONS

- Take command.
- Use track-side telephone (stating the box number and nearest station) to
  alert signalman to warn other trains;
  activate major incident procedure;
  inform of the number of casualties and any other hazard;
  detail the approach route (access in this case is likely to be difficult and casualties and equipment may have to be carried large distances across country).
- Collect the uninjured together so that they may work under your direction.
- Establish a triage area to which casualties can be brought.

With the arrival of further medical assistance one doctor will become Incident Medical Officer (Site Medical Officer) and be responsible for the medical administration: this requires close liason with the Ambulance Incident Officer (and other service incident officers) and the receiving hospitals, and involves setting up a casualty clearing station, calling up extra medical aid and determining the casualty capacity of the receiving hospitals (preferably by direct radio contact).

2. Casualty treatment

		First Aid	**Advanced Life Support**
1st	C* (**P1**)	Open airway (jaw thrust) ensuring on-line traction to the cervical spine with any patient movement. Immobilize cervical spine. Arrest haemorrhage (direct pressure). If using a canvas stretcher to evacuate, do so face down with the forehead supported over the end of the canvas by a bandage between the stretcher poles.	Pull tongue out on a suture (if not supported by floor of mouth). Suction. Cricothyrotomy if above measures fail.
2nd	F (**P1**)	Reassure. Remove the heavy trunk. Support on RIGHT (affected) side and splint flail segment (elastoplast bandage).	Supplemental oxygen at 60% (i.e. 8 litre/minute). If condition is not improved by first-aid measures, or deteriorates, it may be necessary to positive-pressure ventilate: a bystander should be instructed to ventilate at the same rate as their own respirations (otherwise you would be committed to this casualty).
3rd	A (**P1**)	Reassure. Arrest haemorrhage around wound site. Support stake, but **do not** attempt to remove it. Release by cutting stake close to body.	Oxygen, 8 litres/minute. Insert two large intravenous cannulae and restore fluid volume with colloid. Analgesia (morphine). Sample for cross-match to hospital if prolonged extrication *cont.*

---

*Extensive facial trauma has resulted in upper airway obstruction. You should be aware of a possible associated cervical spine injury.

anticipated. MAST suit trousers to maintain blood pressure. Monitor pulse, BP, oxygen saturation (pulse oximeter).

4th H This casualty is shocked. His legs are crushed and
(**P1**) trapped below the knee by twisted metal. Absent pulses indicate the distal limbs are probably inviable. He has a ruptured spleen.

Reassure.
Arrest any accessible point of bleeding.

Oxygen, 8 litres/minute. Establish 2 × i.v.i. and give colloid.
Analgesia (morphine). In view of intra-abdominal injury/inviable distal limbs, amputation is wise to allow speedy extrication. If limbs not amputated, beware hyperkalaemia on release. MAST suit will tamponade limb and intra-abdominal bleeding.

5th D It should be established whether the casualty is a
(**P1**) known epileptic (with an incidental head injury) — ? medalert bracelet — or whether the convulsion is considered secondary to the head injury. In either case, the fitting is likely to stop spontaneously, and time is therefore better spent with other casualties.

First Aid
Ensure patient can not injure himself further during convulsion. Dress scalp wound. When convulsion ceases, place in recovery position.

Advanced Life Support
Nasopharyngeal airway.
Oxygen.
Suction.
Diazemuls if convulsions do not stop spontaneously.

<table>
<tr><td>6th</td><td>E
(**P2**)</td><td colspan="2">This man has a fracture of Cl (atlas) with pressure on the greater occipital nerve. 50% of these will have significant neurological damage.</td></tr>
<tr><td></td><td></td><td>Reassure.
Immobilize cervical spine (improvised collar/sand bags).
Evacuate on stretcher.</td><td>Spinal board or other spinal extrication device.</td></tr>
<tr><td>7th</td><td>B
(**P3**)</td><td>Reassure.
Move away from dead husband.</td><td>Sedate if necessary (phenothiazine/ butyrophenone).</td></tr>
<tr><td>8th</td><td>G
(**P3**)</td><td colspan="2">The animal must take the lowest priority. It is not a doctor's place to treat an injured animal, and particularly you should not administer any drugs, but basic sympathetic care could be expected.</td></tr>
<tr><td></td><td></td><td>Free from panelling.
Dress wound.</td><td>Summon a vet.</td></tr>
</table>

3. Evacuation

1st	F	This casualty's airway is not likely to be satisfactorily managed at the scene.
2nd	H	Life-saving surgery is needed.
3rd	A	Urgent surgery is also required, but this casualty is not as unstable as "H".
4th	C	Once the airway has been secured, it is safe to delay this casualty.
5th	D	If this patient remains unconscious, intracranial haemorrhage needs to be excluded.
6th	E	
7th	B	
8th	G	

The Chemical Incident

A tanker carrying a toxic chemical has jack-knifed and over-turned across two carriageways of a motorway, spilling some of its load. Several cars are also involved. This chemical is volatile, and is absorbed through the skin and mucous membranes producing signs of cholinergic overactivity. The nearest town is 5 km away to the north-east and there is a gentle 3 km/hr south-westerly breeze. You arrive as part of a medical response team from one of the 'stand-by' hospitals and are briefed by the Medical Incident Officer. You will help set up and be working in the casualty clearing station.

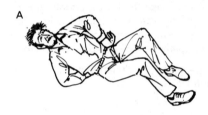

A. Driver of tanker. Unconscious, cyanosed convulsing, constricted pupils.

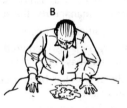

B. Man who helped driver. Laboured breathing and wheeze; rhinorrheoa and sialorrheoa; miosis; muscle twitching; incontinence.

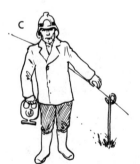

C. Fireman who took his mask off to give mouth-to-mouth. Complaining of blurred vision.

196

D.   Car passenger. Tachycardia,
sweating, tremor, anxious.

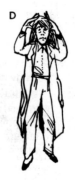

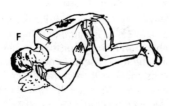

E.   Driver of overturned car.
Pelvis crushed. Pulse 140; blood
pressure 70/? Sweaty and confused.

F.   Found on road near tanker. Reports being splashed by
spilled fluid. Rhinorrheoa, abdominal cramps and vomiting.
Open fracture left forearm.

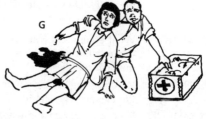

G.   Traumatic amputation right arm at elbow. Scalp
laceration. Pulse 110; blood pressure 100/50.

1. What information will you want to know from the brief?
2. What factors will determine how and where you set up the
    casualty clearing station?

The following casualties arrive as you are still setting up:

3. What is your order of treatment?
4. What is your order of evacuation?

1. Information

You will need to know the following from the brief.

SITUATION	What exactly has happened? (You may not know any details.)
GROUND	What is the layout of the accident and area of immediate hazard? (Should be cordoned off by the police). Are there any important land features (e.g. a steep bank preventing access; marsh excluding site for clearing station)?
AIM	What you have to do.
SAFETY	What protection **you** require to prevent yourself from becoming a casualty (protective suit, gloves overshoes, mask).
CASUALTIES	Estimated numbes of • Chemical casualties • Conventional casualties
HAZARD	What is the chemical? Is it a fire risk (extinguish all sources of ignition) or a vapour hazard? Is it absorbed through, or toxic to, the skin? What are the toxic effects (if not a familiar substance)? Is there a specific antidote and is it available? What are the recommendations for decontamination? (This information is available on the manufacturers Hazard Data Sheet or through the CHEMDATA system, which can be accessed by the fire service).
LOGISTICS	What equipment you have (tents/ decontamination vehicle with shower unit; medical supplies).
SUPPORT	Who is going to help you to set up and operate the clearing station?
COMMAND	Who is in charge and where are they located (incident control)?
SIGNALS	How are you going to communicate? If by radio, determine call-sign and establish radio net.
ROUTES	"Clean" and "dirty" designated routes for contaminated and decontaminated personnel, equipment and vehicles.

You must then brief those under your command.

The need for evacuation of the nearby town is a police decision. Your only concern is the treatment of immediate casualties.

2. Siting the CCS

The casualty clearing station (CCS) must be far enough away from the incident to be remote from a liquid hazard (site uphill if possible), but near enough to avoid casualties needing to be carried large distances. This is particularly important when breathing apparatus is worn, as physical degradation of the stretcher bearers is greatly increased. It may not be possible to be free from a vapour hazard (but site upward and under cover when practicable).

The first priority is to establish a treatment facility, and not to erect tents/decontamination units, so that you are always ready to receive casualties (once your location is known, they will start to arrive whether you are ready or not).

When a chemical that is highly toxic in small amounts is known to be caustic to or can be absorbed through the skin, attempts will have to be made to remove it at the scene. Contaminated clothing can be cut off, sealed in a plastic bag and placed in a contaminated holding area; skin can be washed (showered/sponged) or the chemical adsorbed onto a dry powder. Decontamination is time consuming and some patients will require life-saving intervention first. A canvas stretcher soaked with the diluted chemical is a hazard: cover it with a plastic sheet, or use a synthetic-fibre mesh/scoop stretcher.

3. Casualty Treatment

These chemical effects can be produced by organophosphorus insecticides (e.g. Parathion, Malathion and Metasystox).

1st   B   This is a "chemical immediate" casualty. Do not
     (**P1**)   waste time with decontamination.

First Aid	**Advanced Life Support**
Reassure.	Oxygen plus suction. Give ATROPINE (2 mg i.m./i.v.) and PRALIDOXIME (an enzyme reactivator, 1 g i.m./i.v.). Repeat atropine
	cont.

every 5–10 minutes until breathing eases and secretions reduce (pulse rate is not an accurate measure of adequate atropinization). Repeat pralidoxime after 30 minutes if (in the paralysed) respiration does not improve. Early treatment may avoid the need for ventilatory support. Give Diazemuls for convulsions.

2nd   E
(P1)
This casualty with conventional injuries must also receive intervention before decontamination.

Reassure.	Oxygen.
Lay flat and elevate legs (if pain permits).	Analgesia (splintage; morphine; not likely to co-operate with N_2O). $2 \times$ i.v.i. and rapid volume replacement. MAST suit will stabilize pelvic fracture and help maintain blood pressure.

3rd   F
(P1)
This casualty has moderate poisoning and a conventional injury. It is possible that chemical has contaminated the wound, but upper airway symptoms (rhinorrheoa/sialorrheoa) are commoner with vapour inhalation.

Reassure. Decontaminate wound (copious water) before dressing. Remove contaminated clothing. Splint fracture.	Atropine 2 mg i.m. Pralidoxime 1 g i.m.

4th   G
(P1)

First Aid	**Advanced Life Support**
Direct pressure and elevation to stump. Tourniquet if bleeding not	Oxygen. Analgesia (opiate). Intravenous fluid resuscitation.

controlled (note
time).
Dress scalp wound.

5th   C   This is a mild vapour exposure.
      (P3)

Reassure.   NIL necessary.
Observe for other   Atropine eye drops are
toxic effects.   not effective. The pupils
Decontaminate.   may remain small and
                            vision dim for $1-2$
                            weeks.

6th   D   Many of the symptoms of cholinesterase inhibitor
      (P3) poisoning are the same as ACUTE ANXIETY.

Strongly reassure.   Probably nil — a mild
                            sedative may be
                            necessary.

7th   A   This casualty has severe poisoning. He *may* be
      (Exp.) salvageable: intubate, give oxygen and suction,
            diazemuls, atropine and pralidoxime. Whether he
            is treated first or last will depend on the number
            of trained personnel available to treat other more
            recoverable patients.

4. Evacuation

1st   E
2nd   G
3rd   B   Once treatment has been started for the chemical
            casualties there should be a significant improve-
            ment, and the conventional casualties can take
            priority for evacuation.
4th   F
5th   C
6th   D
7th   A   If it is not anticipated he will survive the journey
            do not use a valuable priority ambulance, BUT
            when you do not have the resources to help,
            urgent evacuation could give the casualty a chance
            of survival.

The Bomb

A bomb has exploded in the street. You are alerted by Ambulance Control and attend the scene within 10 minutes.

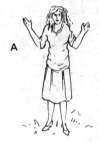

A. Superficial burns to both hands and front of legs below knee.

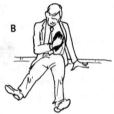

B. Left chest wound; cyanosed; pulse 120; blood pressure 90/40; trachea deviated to right.

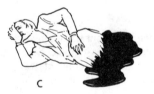

C. Traumatic amputation of lower limbs. No palpable pulse. Slow, gasping respirations.

D. Acutely deaf.

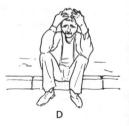

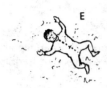

E. Crying baby: no obvious injury.

F. Pregnant woman; multiple facial lacerations. Screaming.

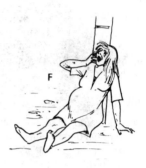

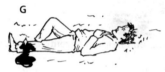

G. Open fracture tibia. Pulse 120; blood pressure 105/80 Dislocated shoulder.

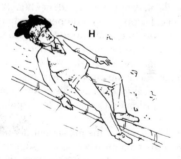

H. Unconscious. Open head injury with exposed brain. Cyanosed. Breathing noisily.

1. What immediate actions will have been taken?
There are the following casualties:

2. What is your order of treatment?

3. What is your order of evacuation?

1. Immediate Actions

SAFETY
Safety is paramount. If not already injured, those in the area are in danger of injury from further explosions. The priorities are:

- **Cordon** — seal the area: this will protect the public and protect the evidence. The immediate area will be evacuated.
- **Search** — look for secondary devices.
- **Isolate** — anything suspicious.

CASUALTIES

- Calculated risks will have to be taken regarding the removal of casualties from immediate further danger and starting life-saving treatment before the area has been cleared.

TRIAGE

- Determine the number and severity of the casualties.

COMMUNICATIONS

- The emergency services are alerted and the Major Incident Plan is activated.
- The Medical/Ambulance Incident Officers will determine the medical support and number of ambulances required at the scene (medical support will usually come from Immediate Care General Practitioners and doctors/nurses from a "stand-by" hospital).
- The main receiving hospital will receive details of the expected number of casualties; the stand-by hospitals should be prepared to take the "overspill" and be alert to self-referring patients.
- The civil police have the initial control of the scene. Help (in the form of manpower, medical support and pyrotechnical expertise) can be requested from the military by the police commander ("Aid to the Civil Authorities" system).
- Press representatives will quickly arrive and, while it is important that information be given out, it is also important that the information, along with the movements of the Press, be controlled.

2. Casualty Treatment

1st B This casualty has a tension pneumothorax.
(P1)

First Aid	Advanced Life Support
He will die if he does not receive definitive care immediately. Direct pressure to chest wound. Place air-tight dressing over wound and hold firm with gauze. Check for exit wound of fragment posteriorly.	Insert large-bore cannula into left 2nd intercostal space: this relieves the tension. Oxygen. Chest drain 4th/5th intercostal space mid-axillary line with Heimlich valve/urine drainage bag (if neither of these are available, use the finger of a rubber glove with a small slit at its tip, tied over the protruding end of the cannula).

2nd G Although the systolic blood pressure is still 105
(P1) mmHg he has a narrow pulse pressure and tachy-cardia, indicative of significant blood loss.

Reassure. Direct pressure and elevation of leg. Splint leg. Broad arm sling.	Oxygen. Analgesia (opiate i.v.). Intravenous fluids. Although it is easier to reduce a dislocated shoulder the earlier it is performed, this is not the place to attempt such a manoeuvre (as the injury is not placing the casualty at any great risk).

3rd D This casualty has been subjected to a significant
(P2) blast effect.

Reassure (may be difficult to communicate). Sit down. Evacuate on stretcher. Observe for respiratory distress.	Oxygen. Ventilatory support if required.

cont.

4th	A (**P2**)	Less than 15% superficial burns.	
		Liberally douse burns with cold water. Plastic bags over the hands and sealed at the wrist are suitable protection.	Analgesia (superficial burns are painful). Intravenous fluids are NOT required. Do not spend time applying dressings and creams — they will be painfully removed in A&E.
5th	F (**P3**)	Reassure.	Nil.
		Arrest bleeding with firm pressure through dressings.	
6th	E (**P3**)	Observe.	If i.v. fluids are subsequently needed but you cannot obtain i.v. access, use an interosseous screw or a needle between the plates of the ilium and halve the flow rate.
		It is probable the baby is unharmed, but will require examination and observation to exclude blast injury. Hand the baby back to the mother — it will distract her from her own suffering.	
7th	H (**Exp**.)	The prognosis of an open head injury is guided by the level of consciousness.	
		Open airway. Dress wound. Place in recovery position on side of wound (provides direct pressure and drainage).	Guedel airway. Withold further intervention until other casualties treated.
8th	C (**Exp**.)	Do not be tempted to try to resuscitate this casualty first — she is going to die. Time spent here may mean patient "B" will also die, unnecessarily.	

3. Evacuation

1st   G

2nd B   This casualty's condition will be sufficiently improved by the insertion of a chest drain to allow the delay in evacuation.

3rd H   G and B must go first although their condition may have improved with treatment all the same, as prolonged delay (for the sake of H) may prove fatal. The prognosis of H is very poor, but he will still take priority over the minor injuries.

4th A   "Blast lung" effects are often not immediately evid-

5th D   ent: if he remains stable at the scene his priority for evacuation will be low.

6th F +E

7th C

Rhythm Sequences

Read the question and look at the rhythm strip.

Decide which of the three responses is the correct treatment.

The answer is given on the following page along with the next rhythm in each series.

RHYTHM SEQUENCE 1

When summoned to a cardiac arrest you witness the following rhythm:

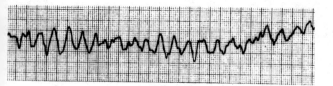

Do you
1. Intubate and then defibrillate?
2. Defibrillate immediately?
3. Give adrenaline 10 ml 1 : 10,000?

Answer: 2

You must defibrillate as early as possible: do not delay to intubate or establish i.v. access at this stage.

Immediately post-defibrillation the monitor displays the following rhythm:

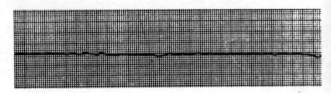

There is no pulse.

Do you

1. Give adrenaline 10 ml 1 : 10,000?
2. Defibrillate again?
3. Give 15 chest compressions and re-check the rhythm?

Answer: 3

Remember, the oscilloscope takes 8–10 seconds to recover.
Check the pulse immediately post-defibrillation — if there is
no pulse palpable, give 15 chest compressions then re-check
the rhythm.
The monitor now reads:

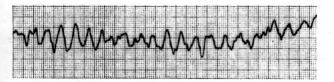

Do you
1. Defibrillate 200 joules?
2. Defibrillate 400 joules?
3. Give lignocaine 100 mg i.v.?

Answer: 1

A second shock of 200 joules may be successful where the first has failed as the transthoracic impedence is reduced by the initial shock.

You need to defibrillate again (400 joules). You then intubate, but are unable to establish i.v. access. The rhythm is:

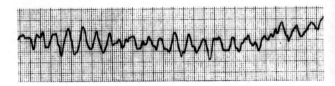

Do you give

1. Adrenaline 10 ml 1 : 10,000 via the endotracheal tube?
2. Adrenaline 20 ml 1 : 10,000 via the endotracheal tube?
3. Adrenaline 10 ml 1 : 10,000 intracardiac?

Answer: 2

Double the dose when giving via the endotracheal tube; do not use the intracardiac route routinely (as drugs rarely reach their intended site and complications are common, including pneumothorax, coronary artery and ventricular laceration and intractable dysrhythmias with intramyocardial injection).

After 2 minutes of chest compression, defibrillation produces the following rhythm:

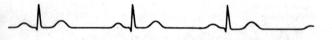

The pulse is palpable.

Do you

1. Just continue to monitor?
2. Start a lignocaine infusion?
3. Start a dobutamine infusion?

Answer: 2

Give lignocaine 4 mg/minute for 30 minutes then 2 mg/minute for 1 hour then 1 mg/minute for the rest of 24 hours to prevent further fibrillation; inotropes such as dobutamine or dopamine would only be necessary if there is additional impaired myocardial contractility.

Despite starting a lignocaine infusion, 10 minutes later the rhythm reverts to:

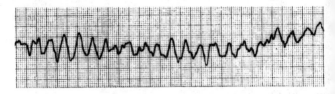

Do you

1. Defibrillate 200 joules?
2. Defibrillate 400 joules?
3. Give NaHCO₃ 50 ml 8.4%?

Answer: 1

The rhythm should be treated as a primary abnormality — i.e. start again at the beginning of the protocol.

Rhythm Sequence 2

A 55-year-old man has collapsed in the street with chest pain. He is in the following cardiac rhythm:

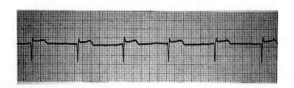

Rate = 55
Blood pressure = 110/60
P–R interval = 0.34 seconds

Do you
1. Give atropine?
2. Give isoprenaline?
3. Observe rhythm?

Answer: 3

This is first-degree heart block (P−R interval > 0.22 seconds). The history and ST elevation suggest acute myocardial infarction. Atropine is only necessary with a bradycardia producing hypotension, pulmonary oedema or syncope. Isoprenaline will increase cardiac rate, but with a risk of inducing ventricular ectopics and tachydysrhythmias — it is not recommended as a chronotrope after myocardial infarction.

You decide to give atropine 0.3 mg i.v. and his rhythm becomes:

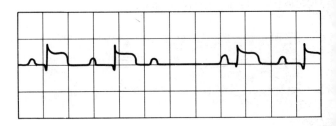

Ventricular rate = 45
Blood pressure = 95/55

Do you

1. Give more atropine?
2. Give physostigmine (atropine antagonist)?
3. Give adrenaline?

This is second-degree heart block, Mobitz Type 1 (Wenkebach phenomenon). Atropine in low doses will occasionally cause transient vagal STIMULATION (a partial agonist, and possibly central, effect).

Atropine 0.6 mg i.v. restores him to sinus rhythm, rate 60 beats per minute. While you are preparing to move the patient to the ambulance, his rhythm changes to:

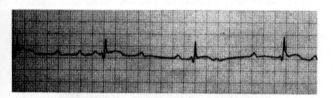

Ventricular rate = 30
Confused and hypotensive

Do you

1. Give chest compressions?
2. Thump the precordium at a rate of 60/minute?
3. Do nothing and transfer to hospital as rapidly as possible?

Answer: 2

This is third-degree, or complete, heart block (with narrow ventricular complexes). Cardiac output can be improved by "fist pacing", i.e. rhythmically thumping the precordium 60 times a minute. Chest compressions are not tolerated if the patient is conscious. A transthoracic pacemaker is an alternative (skin electrodes), although it is uncomfortable (you may need to sedate the patient).

You "fist pace" the casualty. During the journey he loses consciousness and the rhythm is:

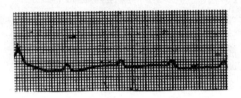

No pulse
You intubate and ventilate

Do you then

1. Give calcium chloride 10 ml 10%?

2. Give atropine 1 mg i.v.?

3. Give adrenaline 10 ml 1 : 10,000?

Answer: 3

Adrenaline is the drug of choice in asystole, to promote spontaneous cardiac contraction.

After 2 minutes chest compression the rhythm is:

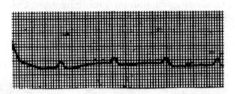

No pulse.

Do you

1. Give adrenaline 10 ml 1 : 10,000?
2. Give atropine 1 mg i.v.?
3. Give bicarbonate 50 ml 8.4% solution?

Answer: 2

Atropine (1–2 mg i.v.) is the second line drug in asystole. Bicarbonate would be considered next. Isoprenaline has not been shown to be useful.

You continue resuscitation for 5 more minutes. On arrival at A&E the rhythm is:

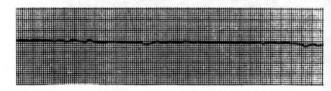

Do you

1. Discontinue resuscitation?
2. Insert a transvenous pacemaker?
3. Give more adrenaline?

Answer: 1

Further resuscitation attempts are unlikely to be successful. Cardiac pacing gives very poor results in asystolic arrest, and would only be considered when there is some electrical activity (i.e. "P" waves).

Rhythm Sequence 3

A 35-year-old woman with known Wolff−Parkinson−White syndrome is complaining of palpitations and shortness of breath for 2 hours. Her ECG shows this rhythm:

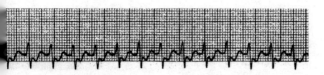

Rate = 180, regular

Do you

1. Give verapamil 5 mg i.v.?
2. Give carotid sinus massage?
3. DC cardiovert 100 joules?

Answer: 2

This is a regular supraventricular tachycardia in Wolff–Parkinson–White syndrome. Measures that decrease A-V conduction are tried before any drugs are considered: carotid sinus massage, Valsalva manoeuvre and an ice-bag over the face ("diving reflex") will all increase vagal tone. Do **NOT** press on the eyeballs — this is not only painful, but can cause retinal detachment.

Carotid sinus massage produces only a temporary slowing of the rate. You give verapamil 5 mg i.v. After 5 minutes the rhythm is:

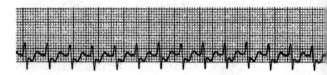

Rate = 180, regular

Do you

1. Give verapamil 5 mg i.v.?
2. Give atenolol 5 mg i.v.?
3. DC cardiovert 100 joules?

Atenolol can be used primarily to terminate supraventricular tachycardia (although verapamil is more commonly used), but it should **NEVER** be given immediately after verapamil as this may result in profound A-V block. Verapamil can be repeated after 5−10 minutes (maximum dose 15−20 mg).

The patient reverts to sinus rhythm. One week later she is again short of breath with dizziness and chest discomfort. Her ECG shows this:

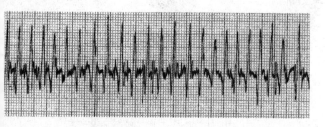

Rate = 220, irregularly irregular
Blood pressure = 100/60

Do you

1. Give verapamil 5 mg i.v.?
2. Give carotid sinus massage?
3. DC cardiovert 100 joules?

Answer: 3

This is atrial fibrillation in Wolff—Parkinson—White syndrome. Inhibiting A-V node conduction can lead to an INCREASE in transmission through the Bundle of Kent and an INCREASE in ventricular rate, which may precipitate ventricular dysrhythmias. Do NOT, therefore, give verapamil (or digoxin). The treatment of choice is to sedate/anaesthetise and cardiovert, starting at a low energy (100 joules); alternatively, disopyramide and sotalol slow conduction through the Bundle of Kent.

You decide to give verapamil 5 mg i.v. which precipitates the following rhythm:

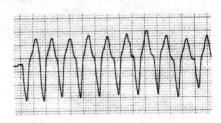

Blood pressure 100/60
Fully conscious

Do you

1. Cardiovert immediately?
2. Give a bolus of lignocaine 100 mg i.v.?
3. Reverse the effect of verapamil with calcium chloride?

Answer: 2

This is ventricular tachycardia. The patient is still well-perfused and it is reasonable to try a bolus of lignocaine, which may be sufficient to terminate the abnormal rhythm. Calcium chloride might improve cardiac output in electromechanical dissociation secondary to calcium antagonist (verapamil) overdose, but would not rectify this ventricular tachycardia.

The patient becomes confused and hypotensive and complains of numbness in her arms. The rhythm is:

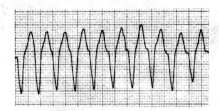

Blood pressure 80/40

Do you

1. Give a second lignocaine bolus?
2. Cardiovert 200 joules?
3. Give procainamide 100 mg i.v.?

Answer: 2

These are common effects of lignocaine toxicity; convulsions can also occur. Her perfusion has deteriorated and she requires cardioversion (under sedation/short acting anaesthetic). Procainamide may work where lignocaine has failed, but is not indicated in this case.

After 200 joules DC cardioversion the rhythm is:

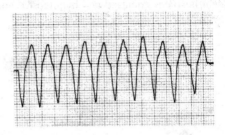

Do you

1. Cardiovert 200 joules?
2. Cardiovert 400 joules?
3. Give bretylium tosylate 5 mg/kg i.v.?

Answer: 1

Ventricular tachycardia producing hypotension or loss of consciousness is treated as ventricular fibrillation. Bretylium tosylate (5 mg/kg bolus followed by 10 mg/kg) is reserved for refractory cases.

A further 200 joules DC cardioversion produces sinus rhythm.

Rhythm Sequence 4

A collapsed patient from a road accident shows the following rhythm on the monitor:

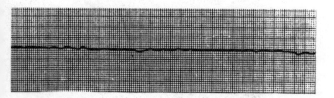

There is no pulse.

Do you

1. Abandon resuscitation?
2. Give adrenaline 10 ml 1 : 10,000?
3. Check the position of the "gain" switch?

Answer: 3

You MUST CHECK the LEADS and the GAIN when the monitor displays "asystole": *do not miss* a potentially treatable dysrhythmia.

You turn up the gain. The following rhythm now appears:

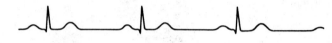

Do you

1. Monitor only?
2. Give calcium chloride 10 ml 10% i.v.?
3. Start basic life support?

Answer: 3

Remember, there was no pulse. This is electro-mechanical dissociation — the likely causes in a trauma victim are tension pneumothorax, cardiac tamponade and hypovolaemia. These should be excluded before any drugs are given (adrenaline is used first).

The neck veins are distended and trachea displaced to the right. You insert a large bore cannula in the second intercostal space on the left. Shortly afterwards, the rhythm is:

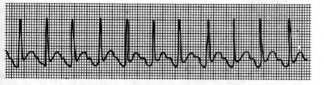

Rate = 135
Blood pressure = 85/50

Do you

1. Try carotid sinus massage?
2. Give fluids intravenously?
3. Give verapamil 5 mg i.v.?

Answer: 2

You have treated the tension pneumothorax (but an elective chest drain is still needed) — electro-mechanical dissociation with distended neck veins suggests tamponade or tension, and with collapsed veins suggests hypovolaemia (not reliable when the two occur together). There is a *sinus* tachycardia. Blood loss must be the first consideration and fluids must be rapidly replaced intravenously.

You give 3 litres of crystalloid over the next 30 minutes and the pulse slows to 90 beats per minute. Three more litres of fluid are given within the next hour. The patient is now breathless and the rhythm is:

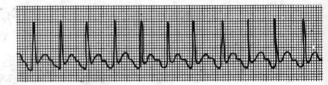

Rate = 110

Do you

1. Give a diuretic?
2. Give more crystalloid?
3. Reinsert the chest drain?

Answer: 1

A blocked chest drain would have to be excluded, but it is more likely this patient has pulmonary oedema resulting from excessive crystalloid (which has a short intravascular half-life).

Ten units of blood are later needed to control delayed catastrophic intra-abdominal bleeding. The ECG trace shows the following abnormality:

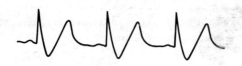

Do you

1. Give 10 ml 10% calcium gluconate?
2. Give 50 ml 50% dextrose + 20 units soluble insulin?
3. Give 4 g KCl over 30 minutes?

Answer: 1+2

"Tented" (tall and peaked) "T" waves, a broad "QRS" and absent "P" waves (because of a nodal rhythm) are all hallmarks of hyperkalaemia. Potassium will leak out of stored red cells with time, but massive transfusion only rarely causes a rise in serum potassium. Warming the blood first will encourage the potassium to return into the cells. Hypocalcaemic tetany is a possibility with a large transfusion of citrated blood but only if given very quickly — this is reversed by intravenous calcium gluconate. Calcium gluconate additionally is cardioprotective in the presence of hyperkalaemia.

References

Adams J.C., *Outline of Fractures*, 9th edn., Churchill Livingstone, Edinburgh, 1987.

American College of Surgeons, *Advanced Trauma Life Support Course* (Student Manual), 1981.

American Heart Association, *Textbook of Advanced Cardiac Life Support*, 1983.

British Association for Immediate Care, *Guide to Major Incident Management*, 1988.

British Association for Immediate Care, *Monographs on Immediate Care* (Numbers 1–5), 1984–87.

Baskett, P. and Weller, R., *Medicine for Disasters*, Wright, London, 1988.

Brown, A.F.T., *Accident and Emergency, Diagnosis and Management*, Heinemann, Oxford, 1988.

Brown, R. And Valman, H., *Practical Neonatal Paediatrics*, 4th edn., Blackwell, Oxford, 1986.

Caroline, N., *Emergency Medical Treatment*, 2nd edn., Little, Brown & Co., Boston, 1987.

Chamberlain, G., *Lecture Notes on Obstetrics*, 5th edn., Blackwell, Oxford, 1984.

Conkin, J.J. and Walker, R.I. (eds.), *Military Radiobiology*, Academic Press, San Diego, 1987.

Dreisbach, R. and Robertson, W., *Handbook of Poisoning*, 12th edn., Lange, Connecticut, 1987.

Evans, R., *Emergency Medicine*, Butterworths, London, 1981.

Evans, T.R. (ed.), *ABC of Resuscitation*, British Medical Association, 1986.

Gandy, G.M. and Roberton, N.R.G., *Lecture Notes on Neonatology*, Blackwell, Oxford, 1987.

Gardiner, P.A., *ABC of Ophthalmology*, British Medical Association, 1979.

Goodman, L. and Gilman, A. (eds.), *The Pharmacological Basis of Therapeutics*, Macmillan, New York, 1980.

Hardy, R., *Accidents and Emergencies*, 4th edn., Oxford University Press, 1985.

Hinds, C.J., *Intensive Care*, Baillière Tindall, London, 1987.

Kelnar, C. and Harvey, D., *The Sick Newborn Baby*, Baillière Tindall, London, 1981.

King, M. (ed.), *Primary Surgery*, Vol. 2, Oxford University Press, 1987.

Kirby, Maj.Gen. N. (ed.), *Field Surgery Pocket Book*, HMSO, London, 1983.

Laurence, D.R. and Bennett, P.N., *Clinical Pharmacology*, 6th edn., Churchill Livingstone, Edinburgh, 1987.

Mather, S.J. and Edbrooke, E., *Prehospital Emergency Care*, Wright, Bristol, 1986.

McGrath, G. and Bowker, M., *Common Psychiatric Emergencies*, Wright, Bristol, 1987.

McRae, R., *Practical Fracture Treatment*, Churchill Livingstone, Edinburgh, 1983.

Page, G. et al., *A Colour Atlas of Cardiopulmonary Resuscitation Techniques*, Wolfe, London, 1986.

Pratt, R., *AIDS — A Strategy for Nursing Care*, 2nd edn., Edward Arnold, London, 1988.

Robinson, R. and Stott, R., *Medical Emergencies, Diagnosis and Management*, 5th edn., Heinemann, London, 1987.

Safar, P. and Bircher, N., *Cardiopulmonary Cerebral Resuscitation*, 3rd end., W.B. Saunders, London, 1988.

Settle, J.A.D., *Burns — The First Five Days*, Smith & Nephew, 1986.

Stoddart, J.C., *Trauma and the Anaesthetist*, Baillière Tindall, London, 1984.

Weatherall, D.J. et al. (eds.), *Oxford Textbook of Medicine*, 2nd edn., Vols. 1 & 2, Oxford University Press, 1987.

Williams, W.G. (ed.), *Trauma of the Chest*, Wright, Bristol, 1977.

Wyngaarden, J. and Smith, L. (eds.), *Cecil, Textbook of Medicine*, 18th edn., W.B. Saunders, London, 1988.